REHABILITATION
OF ARM AMPUTEES AND
LIMB-DEFICIENT
CHILDREN

The author and the publishers have pleasure
in acknowledging the contribution made
by Action Research for the Crippled Child
(the National Fund for Research into Crippling Diseases)
towards the publication of this book

Rehabilitation of Arm Amputees and Limb-Deficient Children

ELIZABETH ROBERTSON

MBAOT

Formerly Senior Occupational Therapist to the Arm Training Unit and Head Occupational Therapist to the Children's Unit, Queen Mary's Hospital, Roehampton, London

with a foreword by

D. S. McKENZIE MB, ChB, FRCS

Formerly Director of the Biomechanical Research and Development Unit, The Limb-fitting Centre, Roehampton, London

BAILLIÈRE TINDALL
LONDON

A BAILLIÈRE TINDALL book published by
Cassell Ltd
35 Red Lion Square, London WC1R 4SG

and at Sydney, Auckland, Toronto, Johannesburg

an affiliate of
Macmillan Publishing Co. Inc.
New York

© 1978 Baillière Tindall
a division of Cassell Ltd

First published 1978

ISBN 0 7020 0714 5

Printed in Great Britain by
Cox & Wyman Ltd, London, Fakenham and Reading

British Library Cataloguing in Publication Data

Robertson, Elizabeth
Rehabilitation of arm amputees and
limb-deficient children.
1. Amputations of arm   2.
Amputees—Rehabilitation   3. Physically
handicapped children—Rehabilitation   4.
Extremities (Anatomy)—Abnormalities
I. Title
362.4'3   RD557

ISBN 0-7020-0714-5

Contents

List of Illustrations

Foreword

It was with very great pleasure that I accepted Elizabeth Robertson's invitation to write a foreword for her book. We were colleagues for many years. She was the pioneer who developed at the Roehampton Limb-fitting Centre the modern techniques of prosthetic training and rehabilitation that are practised today in the United Kingdom and, indeed, through her teachings, in many other countries.

Though the field is numerically small (there are only some 400 new patients admitted to the Limb Service in England and Wales each year) it is very specialized. The patients who suffer arm amputations are predominately young fit adults. The limb deficiencies vary from minor digital defects to total amelia with associated deficiencies of the lower limbs. Life expectancy is long-term and good rehabilitation enhances the quality of that life. Many can be restored to a level where their disability causes scarcely any disablement. Thus the targets for rehabilitation can be set high.

To these Miss Robertson brought her conventional training as an occupational therapist. She also brought a keenly enquiring mind, a shrewd instinct for what is biomechanically viable and above all total clinical honesty. She was quick to recognize the critical importance of early contact with the patient—within days for amputees and as soon as possible after birth for the limb-deficient children. At this stage counselling based on early assessment is given. Prosthetic fitting when indicated is undertaken at the earliest possible moment to counteract the inherent tendency to one-handed function. The programme of rehabilitation is planned and explained and a reasoned prognosis can be given. Miss Robertson also appreciates that she was treating not just an amputation stump, not just a limb with a congenital deficiency, but a whole patient, a whole child, the parents, the environment to which the patient will return and all the other factors which infringe on rehabilitation.

In her book, Miss Robertson's description of general management and of prostheses available follow the accepted UK practice. It is when she comes to dealing with the specific role of the therapist that the book becomes alive. Here speaks the authority of a unique experience coupled with acute observation and interpretation. I can confidently recommend the book as required reading for all those concerned with the management of this small but important group of patients.

January 1978   D. S. McKenzie

Preface

Limbs have been amputated and children have been born with all or part of limbs missing since the beginning of time. Replacement of a leg and learning to walk with an artificial limb has always taken priority over the rehabilitation of those people with all or part of an arm missing. Until the twentieth century most upper limb prostheses were designed with the idea of completing the body with a limb that looked as lifelike as possible, with little attention being paid to the usefulness of the prosthesis. When a functional prosthesis was provided it was usually only a simple hook for which little training was available or necessary. Although more sophisticated upper limb prostheses were available in the early part of this century it was not until the early 1940s that an arm training school was set up at Roehampton to train service personnel to make the maximum use of their artificial arms. In 1948 when the National Health Service made it possible for all United Kingdom residents to be supplied free with all necessary prostheses, the training facilities were expanded to provide a national service for civilians. Although limb-deficient children were then eligible, it was several more years before these children were being routinely fitted at a young enough age for them to have a reasonable chance of learning to use a prosthesis in a natural manner.

The realization that the acceptance and use of an arm prosthesis depends not only on the physical ability to control the prosthesis, but also on the establishment of neurological patterns of bimanual arm use, has led those working in the field of prosthetics to the belief that the time without a functional limb must be kept to a minimum. This has meant that the rehabilitation of arm amputees and limb-deficient children is no longer the prerogative of the prosthetics services but must start as soon as the limb is lost or the child is born.

This book endeavours to describe the stages of this rehabilitation so that those people suddenly faced with the problem of an amputee or limb-deficient child among their patients or acquaintances can have some idea of what the future holds for him. Although much of the book is in the form of a handbook for those professionally involved in the training of arm amputees and limb-deficient children, there is much that should be helpful to amputees, their families and their friends. Because the attitude of the limb-deficient person towards the absence of an arm influences his rehabilitation, it is vitally important that all those concerned should understand his present and future problems and be aware of how they can help him adjust to his loss.

The book is divided into four sections. The first part describes the early rehabilitation from the time the amputee loses his arm, or the limb-deficient child is born, to his referral to the limb-fitting service. Much of the rehabilitation at this stage can be carried out by the hospital staff who are readily available, although the participation of someone who has some knowledge of prosthetics and the training of arm amputees is helpful. The second part provides an introduction to upper limb prosthetics, describing their history, the different types of prostheses and terminal devices available and how they are controlled. The importance of early fitting of prostheses is discussed here and the various types of temporary prostheses described. The detailed training of the adult arm amputee with his prosthesis is the subject of part three. The three stages of training are described; control of the prostheses, use of the prosthesis in bimanual activities and application of this training to the amputee's job, hobbies and everyday life. The final part of the book is devoted to the child amputee and the limb-deficient child. It starts by discussing the appropriateness of prostheses for some of these children. Because it has been shown that many limb-deficient children achieve more without, rather than with, prostheses, much of this section is devoted to ways of helping them make maximum use of their residual abilities.

Throughout the book an attempt has been made to emphasize that the best solution for each arm amputee and limb-deficient child is the one that suits that individual. There are no hard-and-fast rules in this relatively new field of rehabilitation. We are only recently seeing the results of the principle of early fitting of prostheses to limb-deficient children and beginning to analyse why it works for some and not for others. The same is true of immediate postoperative fitting and training of adults. I feel strongly that too often arm prosthetics have not been given a fair chance; that equipment has been declared useless when it is fitting and training that have been inadequate. Nobody is going to wear and use an uncomfortable prosthesis when it is not essential to his existence. The pressure on the amputee to take action about an ill-fitting lower limb prosthesis is infinitely greater than for an upper limb. The arm amputee is unaware of the potential of his prosthesis until he has been taught to use it. Learning to operate the controls is not enough to ensure that the majority of arm amputees learn to use their prosthesis efficiently. The principles behind its function are often alien to the natural method of achievement and unless he is taught how to control and make use of his prosthesis he will either discard it or wear it for purely dress purposes.

The fitting of limb-deficient children with prostheses has in the past been coupled with the fitting of arm amputees. Superficially their problems may look the same but in fact they are very different. It is hoped that this difference has been made clear in the last part of this book and that perhaps it may influence those involved with the management of these children to think again before advocating prostheses in every case.

July 1978   ELIZABETH ROBERTSON

Acknowledgements

There have been many people who have provided help and encouragement with this book. I am grateful to all of them and wish to thank them sincerely for their contributions. Many must remain anonymous, but special reference must be made to the following: Miss J. Mendez OBE, Group Head Occupational Therapist at Queen Mary's Hospital, Roehampton, who not only encouraged me but also provided practical help with the planning and writing of the book; Dr D. S. McKenzie, who gave me access to the available literature and supported my efforts by writing the Foreword; Clare Singer for her excellent line drawings; and my sisters for their unfailing help and encouragement. Dr I. Fletcher and the Department of Medical Illustration at Queen Mary's Hospital generously supplied many of the photographs and the Medical Superintendent of Groote Schuur Hospital, Cape Town, kindly gave his permission to reproduce the illustrations of the Dynamic Enabler. Last but not least I would like to thank all those arm amputees, limb-deficient children and their families from whom I have learned so much.

E.R.

PART I

Early Stages in Rehabilitation

CHAPTER 1

The Team Approach

The loss of a limb is a profound shock to an individual and for parents to have a child with all or a part of a limb missing is a tragedy which is hard for them to bear. Yet they must accept it with all its implications if they are to benefit from the help available. If they remain resentful, or feel guilty about what has happened, rehabilitation will be more difficult. It is right that all amputees feel grief and mourn the loss or absence of a limb, but mourning must come to an end if the best of life is to continue. Determination is going to be needed to succeed with what may be a handicap but usually need not be a disability.

Many people are concerned in the rehabilitation of the amputee, each with a part to play in helping him to adjust to the loss of his limb. If they are to be successful they should be familiar with the other aspects of the amputee's rehabilitation as well as their own specialty.

This book will endeavour to provide an outline of the arm amputee's rehabilitation, with special emphasis on his pre-prosthetic and prosthetic training. It also describes the training of limb–deficient children, with information on aids and adaptations developed in various centres to help them achieve their full potential.

Arm amputees and limb-deficient children may receive their pre-prosthetic treatment and training in the use of their prosthesis in a hospital, a rehabilitation centre, an arm training unit in a limb-fitting centre or, in the case of some children, in a regional assessment centre or a special school. Wherever training is carried out the principles are the same and the therapist is part of a team which may extend beyond her hospital, centre or school. This team has at its centre the patient, cared for by his family, doctor, nurse, social worker, physiotherapist, occupational therapist, limb-fitting surgeon and prosthetist. Other experts such as the engineer, research worker, teacher, disablement resettlement officer and employers will also be involved, but not for every patient. In the early stages the surgeon and the nurse will be of primary importance, with the social worker assisting. At the pre-prosthetic stage the physiotherapist and then the occupational therapist have a more important role to play. When the amputee is referred to the limb-fitting centre, the limb-fitting surgeon and the prosthetist with his colleagues in the factory become the pivot of the rehabilitation team, with the occupational therapist, physiotherapist and nurse giving supporting services. Finally when the amputee has his prosthesis the therapist becomes the most involved in the training programme. Throughout the family is of prime importance in encouraging and supporting the amputee.

Only when individual members of the team understand the whole process of the amputee's rehabilitation can they know when to take a leading role in this rehabilitation and when to provide a secondary or supporting service. Arm amputees are not common in a general hospital nor is a baby often born with part of a limb missing. These are rare occurrences and so are a challenge to the staff involved. Each team member must identify his role and offer his skills at the appropriate time.

CHAPTER 2

Amputation and Immediate Postoperative Treatment

The majority of upper limb amputees lose an arm as the result of an accident. They usually lose one arm, either below or above the elbow. A much smaller number have their arm amputated because of disease and these are more likely to be above-elbow, through-shoulder or forequarter amputations because of the necessity to amputate well above the diseased part of the limb. A very few upper limb amputees lose one or both arms as the result of cardiovascular insufficiency. Double arm amputations are almost always the result of an accident and fortunately do not occur often. Following trauma the surgeon frequently has little choice in selecting the site of amputation. The general rule is to preserve length but sometimes this can cause problems later when fitting the prosthesis. A brief study of the prostheses available and their mechanics will explain why.

If an above-elbow prosthesis is to be cosmetically acceptable as well as functional it must have a joint at the elbow. If the amputation is through the elbow the mechanical joint of the prosthesis has to be in the form of external side steels which are bulky and catch in clothes. It is therefore preferable that the amputation should be sufficiently far above the elbow joint (approximately two-thirds of the humeral length) to allow the elbow mechanism to be housed within the upper arm of the prosthesis. A slightly different situation arises with amputations at wrist level, for a through-wrist amputation retains active wrist rotation, a movement which cannot at present be replaced in a body-powered prosthesis. But should it be necessary to amputate above the distal end of radius it is better to shorten the stump sufficiently to allow the prosthetic forearm to be the same length as the normal arm after the wrist unit has been incorporated into the prosthesis.

Because of the traumatic nature of most arm amputations it is usually not possible to prepare patients for amputation. It is unlikely that they have ever considered losing a limb or have even known an arm amputee. It is a tremendous shock to them and may seem quite unbelievable for several days. They may still be able to feel their arm (phantom limb) and imagine that they are moving their fingers. This makes it seem even more unreal. They should be encouraged to look at and to handle their stumps as early as possible to help them become accustomed to the fact of having lost a limb. One of the easiest ways to do this is to encourage patients to wash their own stumps and to help with dressings and bandaging.

They should start to use their stumps for leaning on and for steadying objects as soon as postoperative tenderness has subsided. Within a few days they can start simple resisted exercises to maintain the tone in muscles proximal to the amputation and to ensure that no joint movement is lost. Particular emphasis should be placed on exercises to build up triceps in the below-elbow amputee and pectoralis major and deltoid in the above-elbow amputee, as these muscles play an active role in operating the prosthesis. The whole scapula should be kept mobile. The handling of the stump necessary to do these exercises will further help them to come to terms with their amputation and make them realize that a stump is not just a useless remnant of a limb.

At this stage arm amputees can very easily feel that their life is finished and that they will no longer be able to earn a decent living or take part in their favourite sports and hobbies. They will feel incomplete and an object of pity to their friends and relatives. Realistic discussion of their future abilities and prospects can often be helpful, but care must be taken not to encourage them to think that an artificial arm will look and feel like a real arm. Many amputees arrive at the limb-fitting centre expecting to get a new arm as good as the one that they have lost. When they see their prosthesis they are then bitterly disappointed and find it difficult to accept.

CHAPTER 3

Bandaging

A freshly amputated stump must be bandaged at all times with an elasticated bandage. This should be started as soon as the stitches are removed or when advised by the doctor. Bandaging helps to control oedema and to condition the stump for limb wearing. A 7 cm (3 in) bandage should be used for all arm stumps, except on a small child when a 5 cm (2 in) width may be more practical. It must be applied correctly if it is to serve its purpose: pressure should be applied distally to proximal to assist venous return and the bandage should be firm but not too tight. It should be re-applied at least twice a day and more frequently if the patient is making active use of the stump. Always remove and re-apply the bandage if the stump becomes cold or painful. Bandages should be washed and rinsed frequently using warm (not hot) water. Winding around a line to dry will help to preserve their elasticity. Suitable bandages are available for amputees at the limb-fitting centre.

Although the principles of stump bandaging are the same for all amputations the method varies slightly at different levels in order to give a satisfactory result.

Below-elbow (Fig. 1)

The bandage is taken from the front over the end of the stump to just below the elbow at the back (1); this is then held in position with the index finger and thumb of the left hand while taking the bandage twice more over the end of the stump slightly to each side of the original turn (2 and 3). There are now three thicknesses over the end of the stump.

Diagonal bandaging is then started with minimal stretch on the downwards turns (4) and half-stretch on the upwards turns (5). Tension on the bandage should decrease as it proceeds up the arm to the elbow with sufficient turns to cover the stump adequately.

7

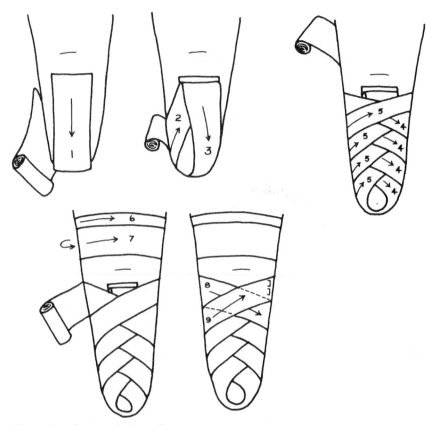

Fig. 1. Bandaging a below-elbow stump.

When the stump is short the bandage should be taken behind and to the side of the olecranon and twice round the upper arm, taking care not to restrict the elbow movement (6 and 7). It should then be brought round the opposite side of the olecranon to below the elbow and completed with two diagonal turns around the forearm (8 and 9). On longer stumps it is not always necessary to take the bandage above the elbow and if it feels secure it can be finished off below.

Above-elbow (Fig. 2)

The bandage is taken from the front, just below the shoulder joint, over the end of the stump to a similar level at the back (1). While holding this with the index finger and thumb of the left hand, bring the bandage twice more over the end of the stump slightly to each side of the original turn finishing at the back (2 and 3).

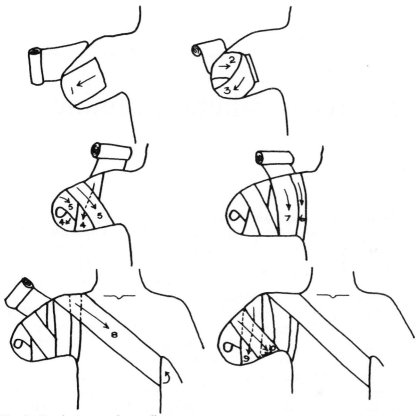

Fig. 2. Bandaging an above-elbow stump.

Start the diagonal turns by coming over the top of the stump and down to the end of the stump at the front (4) passing under and then over the end (5). Continue diagonal bandaging until the stump is adequately covered, with decreasing tension as the bandage gets near the axilla. Make sure that the bandage is taken right into the axilla, with two turns over the point of the shoulder (6 and 7). This is to prevent a roll of flesh developing above the bandage which would be uncomfortable when wearing a prosthesis.

For the long above-elbow the bandage can then be finished off with two more diagonal turns around the stump (9 and 10). To keep the bandage securely in place on a short stump it is necessary to take a turn around the body under the opposite arm (8) before finishing off with the two diagonal turns around the stump (9 and 10). Care must be taken not to restrict the movement of the shoulder when taking the bandage round the body.

9

CHAPTER 4

Pre-prosthetic Training

Training towards using an artificial arm starts as soon as the amputee regains consciousness, or before if it is an elective amputation. If the patient is to make full use of his prosthesis it is vitally important that he accepts the loss of his limb and is not resentful. He needs someone to discuss this with and the social worker, occupational therapist or physiotherapist will often be the person he turns to. She should be able to explain what his abilities and limitations will be with a prosthesis and encourage him to think in terms of independent living. It is important that he retains the idea of being two-handed. He may have to alter the way that he tackles various activities or change his dominance, but once he starts to think in terms of doing everything with his one remaining hand the death knell has sounded for good functional use of his prosthesis. Time spent listening to and talking with a patient at this stage is time well spent, for the more the amputee understands his amputation the easier will be his rehabilitation.

An arm without a hand appears to most people a useless remnant of a limb. The amputee must be convinced that this is not so. Many activities can be adapted so that he uses his stump in a meaningful way. They will depend on his interests and aptitudes as well as his dominance and the length of his stump and many will also have additional value as treatments. They will improve circulation and this in turn will help to heal the stump and control postoperative oedema. They will maintain and stimulate normal neurophysiological patterns of movement and, if properly structured, maintain and improve muscle tone and range of movement proximal to the site of amputation. At first activities must be carefully graded, as the patients are expecting to fail. It must be remembered that they are being asked to do fine skills with muscles which are designed for gross unskilled movements, so treatment periods should be kept short to prevent undue physical and mental fatigue.

The arm amputee should continue with some of these activities until he receives his artificial arm, otherwise he will quickly lose muscle tone and his normal neurophysiological patterns of movement. The development of one-handedness is the biggest handicap to single arm amputees becoming good prosthetic users. This is particularly liable to happen if the non-dominant hand has been lost. Ideally the amputee should continue to attend his parent hospital for treatment until he receives his prosthesis. If this is not possible the physiotherapist and the occupational therapist should make sure that he understands the importance of continuing to exercise and use his stump and that he has a programme of exercises and activities to continue with at home.

Exercises and activities

BELOW-ELBOW

Non-dominant arm

1. Holding down objects while cutting, pasting, drawing, folding, sanding, sawing, planing, or sewing on a machine, to show the amputee that his stump is useful and to encourage two-handedness.
2. Typing with a rubber-tipped peg strapped to the stump: start with the space bar, then the shift lock and finally half the keys with the amputated arm. This activity has several treatment values as it builds up muscle tone, de-sensitizes the stump, assists in learning fine control of shoulder and elbow muscles and in recognition of the position in space of the stump end and reinforces the normal neurophysiological patterns of movement.
3. Bimanual activities using a leather gauntlet (Fig. 3), strapped firmly around the stump over the elasticated bandage, into which various tools with long handles can be inserted, i.e. dish mop, knife for cutting food, knitting needle.

Dominant arm

Use exercises 1, 2 and 3 as for the non-dominant arm. In addition:

4. Unilateral activities normally done with the dominant hand such as painting or varnishing with the brush inserted in the gauntlet and table tennis with the bat similarly fixed.
5. Drawing and writing with a soft pencil or nylon-tipped pen inserted in the gauntlet at an appropriate angle. Ball-point pens should be avoided as they do not provide sufficient friction, as should hard pencils and crayons as they require too much pressure (wax crayons

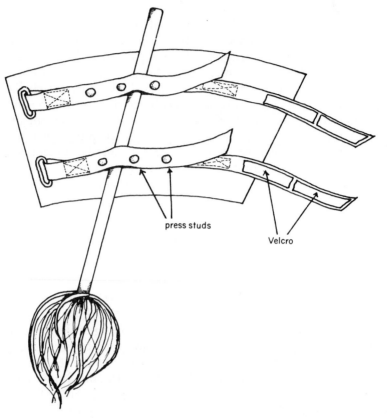

press studs

Velcro

Fig. 3. A gauntlet for pre-prosthetic activities.

can be used but are inclined to break). Before writing is attempted writing patterns (Richardson 1935) should be drawn on plain paper to encourage a smooth even control of the pencil. As the patterns become smaller and more controlled a single line can be introduced. Double lines should be avoided as these cause tension, leading to uneven formation of shapes and letters. Drawing and word games help to maintain interest. The artistic enjoy painting and sketching and for the non-artistic painting by numbers is suitable. About 50% of amputees who lose their dominant arm below the elbow find it easier to learn to write with their prosthesis rather than change to their non-dominant hand. This is particularly true of people who write a great deal in the course of their work or hobby, i.e. teachers, clerical workers, storemen.

6. Activities to improve the skill of the remaining non-dominant hand. Most activities involving the manipulation of an object within

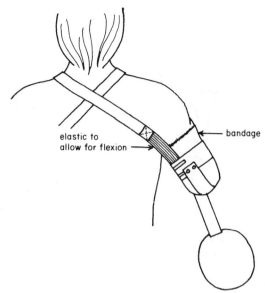

elastic to
allow for flexion →

bandage

Fig. 4. A gauntlet for playing table tennis.

the hand will be more easily done by the remaining non-dominant hand, i.e. handling money, striking a match, hand sewing, fastening buttons, using scissors, shaving or applying cosmetics.

ABOVE-ELBOW

1. Holding objects steady is often difficult because of the shortness of the stump in relation to the other arm. This inequality of length can be overcome by using a rubber-tipped peg in a gauntlet, but the range of suitable activities is more limited. Sanding, sawing and planing are not usually suitable because the amputee is unable to maintain sufficient pressure on the object.

2. Typing. It may be necessary to do this as a practice activity for the stump rather than as a bimanual activity. Place the typewriter on a high table slightly angled towards the amputated side and type for short periods using the stump only.

3. Bimanual activities using a gauntlet. The practicality of these will depend on the length of the stump; if they can be carried out they are a valuable part of treatment as they help to maintain the idea of two-handedness.

4. Unilateral activities for the dominant stump. Painting and table tennis are both practical for the above-elbow amputee. A special gauntlet (Fig. 4) for a table tennis bat can be fabricated for quite a short

13

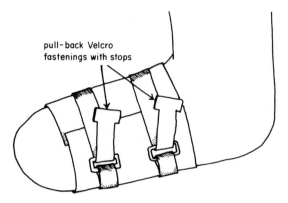

Fig. 5. A gauntlet for the double arm amputee.

stump. This activity is particularly recommended as it demands forward flexion of the stump (the movement that is required to activate the prosthesis).

5. Drawing and writing should be practised when the dominant arm is lost as a few above-elbow amputees find this easier than changing to their non-dominant hand and with proper structuring it can provide valuable exercise for the stump. It is best done on a surface with a tilt of 45° or more to encourage forward flexion of the stump. Writing should be kept large and fine skill not expected. Most above-elbow amputees find it easier to learn to write with their non-dominant hand.

6. Activities to improve the skill of the remaining non-dominant hand are even more important for the above-elbow than for the below-elbow amputee as he will depend to a greater degree on this hand. Time should be spent practising writing with the non-dominant hand.

DOUBLE ARM AMPUTEES

The double arm amputee must be shown as soon as possible that he is not helpless and that he will be able to lead a useful and independent life. Immediate success is needed. This can then be followed by other activities requiring more practice. At this stage many activities will require one or two gauntlets. These should be made with pull-back Velcro fastenings and stops to prevent the straps coming out of the rings (Fig. 5). A suggested order of presenting activities is as follows:

1. Drawing, painting and writing, with emphasis on the first two for practice in control, although writing will prove the greater morale booster. Few people realize that fluent writing is a mental activity and

can be done quite well with the arm and shoulder girdle and not the hand. Writing should be done with the dominant stump unless the non-dominant stump is appreciably longer, i.e. dominant above-elbow with non-dominant below-elbow. In this case writing should be tried with both arms, allowing the patient to choose which he finds easier as it will depend on the strength of the individual's dominance. The method of using writing and drawing as a treatment medium is the same as for the single arm amputee. The paper will have to be stabilized by placing it on a sheet of pimple rubber used the wrong way up, thin Dycem sheeting or some other thin non-slip material (Dycem mats or latex mesh are not suitable). Alternatively secure the paper to a board with thumb tacks, sticky tape or bull-dog clips.

2. Typing with one or both stumps, depending on their length and sensitivity, using a similar method to that for the single arm amputee. For some double arm amputees this may eventually take the place of writing.

3. Self-feeding. Bent cutlery or a self-righting spoon (see Fig. 49) may be necessary for the double above-elbow amputee. A plate guard (see Fig. 38) and non-slip mat may help in the early stages.

4. Toilet independence. Although this is much more difficult to achieve it should be attempted if at least one stump is below-elbow.

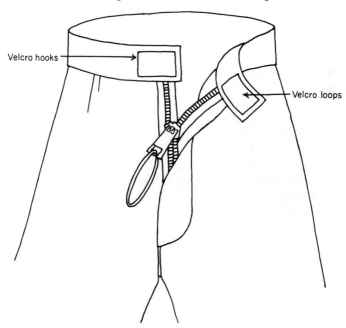

Velcro hooks

Velcro loops

Fig. 6. A modification of the trouser fastening for a double arm amputee.

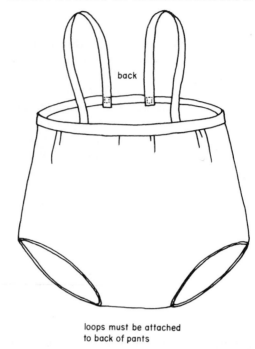

loops must be attached
to back of pants

Fig. 7. A modification to the pants for a double arm amputee.

Modifications to clothing will probably be necessary. The most likely of these are a loop, long enough to insert the stump in, on the fly zip with Velcro waist fastening for men (Fig. 6), and for women loops on pants (Fig. 7) which should be loose fitting and of cotton or jersey material. Careful choice of garments can often obviate alterations, i.e. all garments should be loose fitting; men will find boxer underpants easier than Y-fronts; women often find slacks with elastic at the waist, which can be pulled down with the feet or fastened at the front like men's trousers, easier to manage than skirts. Pants can be fastened inside trousers with large press-studs to halve the effort involved. The young and agile double arm amputee may be able to learn to use toilet paper in the way described for limb-deficient children in Chapter 17. Otherwise this should be left until the amputee has his prosthesis.

5. Bathing is an activity which will always be done without prostheses, so it is as well to start practising at an early stage. A towelling mitt made to fit over the longer stump is useful when used with an octopus soap holder to prevent the soap from slipping; alternatively a pocket for the soap can be made in the towelling mitt (Fig. 8). For washing the back, feet and perineum a long flannel with pockets either end, into which the stumps can be slipped, may prove satisfactory

16

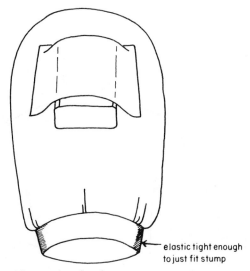

elastic tight enough
to just fit stump

Fig. 8. A towelling mitt with a pocket for the soap.

(Fig. 9), or a long flannel with loops either end (available commercially as Long John Flannels) can be used by hooking one end over the tap. Drying may be made easier by using a roller towel with an elastic loop. When the loop is hung over a hook at shoulder level it is possible to get inside the towel (see Fig. 64) or put one arm into it and turn to dry the back (Fig. 10); elastic loops are better than tape as they allow some give and so are less likely to be ripped off. A wall electric fire or fan heater in

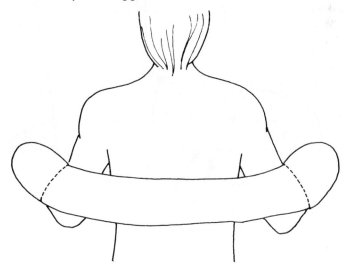

Fig. 9. A long flannel, with pockets at either end, for washing the back.

17

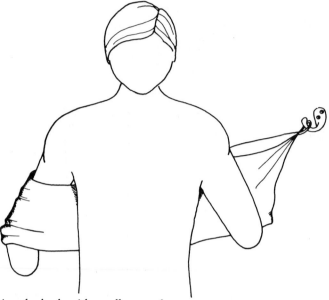

Fig. 10. Drying the back with a roller towel.

the bathroom is a great help to a double arm amputee as there are often small areas of his body that he is unable to reach.

6. Independence in specific activities of importance to an individual can often be tackled satisfactorily at this stage. For the smoker it is

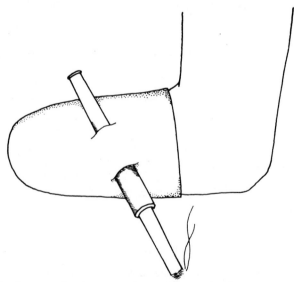

Fig. 11. A plaster socket incorporating a cigarette-holder.

18

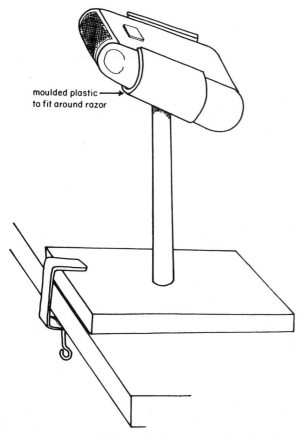

moulded plastic ──➤
to fit around razor

Fig. 12. A razor on a stand which can be clamped to the edge of the table.

usually possible to attach a cigarette holder to a strap or a plaster socket (Fig. 11); he can then take the cigarette out of the packet with his lips, place it on the table, insert it in the holder steadied with the other stump. Shaving is usually easier if an electric or battery razor is fixed to a stand which can then be clamped to a high table (Fig. 12). The amputee can then move his chin on the razor. Women should choose their cosmetics so that they can be held either between their stumps or in a gauntlet, i.e. stick eye shadow and mascara. Both face-powder and talcum can be applied with a puff on a handle made from sheepskin wrapped around a dowel.

References

Richardson, M. (1935) *Writing Patterns*, Book 1. London: University of London Press.

CHAPTER 5

The Limb-deficient Child

The first thing that most mothers ask when their baby is born is whether he has all his fingers and toes. The vast majority of doctors and midwives can joyfully answer 'Yes'. A very few are suddenly faced with the unexpected and difficult task of saying 'No'. That many find the task impossible is not surprising, but none the less tragic, as so much depends on the answer to that first question. It is usually better to tell the truth at once. If a spontaneous and convincing answer is not given the mother will know that there is something wrong and imagine far worse than the facts. It is most unlikely that the baby will have more than one hand or foot missing or deformed. Deficiencies as extensive as those seen during the thalidomide episode do occur, but are very rare.

Once the parents have recovered from the initial shock they will want to talk to someone who can reassure them about the baby's future. This must be a person who is able to offer positive information as well as a sympathetic ear. He or she must know what artificial limbs are available and be able to explain to the parents how they can be referred to a limb-fitting centre for advice. The parents will then have something positive to do towards their baby's future.

The baby will not need an artificial limb until he is several months old nor training until he is older, but the parents need help to adjust to their baby's deficiency. The sooner they are referred to a limb-fitting centre the better, for the isolation and despair of a family with such a child is hard to describe and will be considerably eased if they can be given some idea of what the future holds, and have the opportunity to meet other families in a similar predicament (*Lancet*, 1973). In the meantime the social worker should maintain contact with the parents to help them overcome the difficult transition from hospital to home with a handicapped child. A practical suggestion which some parents who have a baby with one hand missing find helpful is to sew a stuffed mitten to the end of the baby's coat sleeve when they take him out. This can prevent the stares and comments of strangers which are very distressing to parents at a highly emotional time. At home they should be encouraged to leave the stump uncovered so that the baby can learn by touch and develop a body image and bilateral patterns of movement.

If the baby has more than one hand or foot missing he may need practical help before the provision of artificial limbs. He could need a sitting support if both legs are severely affected; if both arms are deficient the parents will need advice on how to encourage play activities and self-feeding. Sometimes children who have more severe deformities are referred directly to a special children's unit associated with a limb-fitting centre where they can be admitted with their mother for several days' assessment. This also gives the mother the opportunity to meet the team who will be involved in their child's future training and to meet other parents and children with similar handicaps. Seeing how well a limb-deficient child and his family manage is often more helpful than advice from professionals.

References

Lancet (1973) Having a congenitally deformed baby. *Lancet*, i, 1499.

CHAPTER 6

The Limb-fitting Service in the United Kingdom

In recent years various reports (British Orthopaedic Association 1973) have described the organization and scope of the limb-fitting service in Britain, but little has been written explaining to the amputee what to expect on his first and subsequent visits to a limb-fitting centre.

The amputee will be referred to the limb-fitting centre by either his surgeon or his general practitioner. This should be as soon as possible after amputation and in the case of an elective amputation it should be before. This will apply to a minority of upper limb amputees and the majority of lower limb amputees. In special cases a limb-fitting surgeon might visit a patient in hospital but the more normal practice is for the patient to attend the limb-fitting centre as an out-patient.

The purpose of this first visit is for the limb-fitting surgeon to meet the amputee and to examine his stump to assess whether it is ready to be measured for a prosthesis. If it is, he will discuss with the patient and the other members of the clinical team the type of prosthesis which would be most suitable, bearing in mind the amputee's age, sex, physique, occupation and hobbies. If a prosthesis is to be ordered at once the amputee will be referred to the prosthetist for casts and measurements to be taken. Alternatively he could be provided with a temporary prosthesis or be referred back to his parent hospital for further treatment, with a subsequent appointment at the limb-fitting centre. He may meet other members of the limb-fitting team such as the nurse, social worker, occupational therapist and physiotherapist if their skills are needed at that stage. He should leave the centre with some idea of what his future programme is to be.

Once the patient has been measured for his prosthesis, it will take several weeks to manufacture and during this time it may be necessary for the amputee to return to the limb-fitting centre for a fitting. When he has received his limb, he will again see the limb-fitting surgeon so that he can check that the limb is satisfactory. Unless training has already started with a temporary prosthesis it will be recommended at this stage. It may be necessary for the amputee to travel to another hospital or centre for training and this should have been explained to him on his first visit to the centre.

During the first year after amputation the patient will receive regular appointments to attend the limb-fitting centre. It is important that he do so. At this stage his stump can change shape so that his prosthesis becomes a poor fit. It is then liable to cause abrasions and become difficult to use. If this is attended to at once no harm will be done; if left, the amputee will tend to discard his prosthesis as a useless, uncomfortable encumbrance. Once the stump has settled into its final shape a duplicate limb will be ordered; when this is completed the original prosthesis can, if necessary, be refitted and serve as a spare limb should the other one have to be sent away for repairs. A broken prosthesis should always be returned to the limb-fitting centre promptly for repairs, otherwise the amputee could find himself with both limbs out of order.

When the amputee has his two prostheses both fitting well and comfortable, it should not be necessary for him to attend the limb-fitting centre regularly. Contact should be maintained, however, and he will receive regular postal communications, usually yearly, enquiring as to the state of his prosthesis and stump and offering to make an appointment if this is needed. It is not necessary for him to wait for one of these letters. He can, at any time, contact his nearest limb-fitting centre for an appointment even if this is not the one which he previously attended. He should not hesitate to do this if at any time his prosthesis becomes unsatisfactory. Should his circumstances change and demand new skills he may need further training; this sometimes happens when a new job is envisaged, retirement approaches or a marriage partner becomes incapacitated. Further training can be arranged at any time by the limb-fitting surgeon.

Children are seen regularly throughout their growing years so that their prostheses can be adjusted to their growth. When children are growing fast it is not always possible for them to have a spare prosthesis which fits them well. The usual practice is for them to have one limb which is a good fit and the correct length with the previous limb as a spare which would do in an emergency. Children will need short periods of training throughout their childhood as their prosthesis becomes more sophisticated and their needs change. Regular contact between the therapist, the child and his parents and the limb-fitting surgeon should enable these to be fitted in to coincide with other appointments or in school holidays.

The amputee will be provided with stump socks from the limb-fitting stores. These should be washed regularly and always if they have become damp with perspiration. If they are not and are allowed to dry and be worn again, the salts in perspiration will harden them. This can cause inflamed areas on the skin of the stump. The normal allocation is 12 socks per stump for a year; these may be of wool, cotton or nylon depending on the individual's requirements. The limb-fitting stores also hold stocks of elasticated bandages, walking sticks, crutches, rubber ferrules and certain appliances for arm amputees. Some of these can only be issued on the doctor's prescription.

There are limb-fitting centres all over Britain, so no patient who needs straightforward limb fitting need travel far for this service. Those with special problems may need to be referred to one of the major centres. This also applies to training in the use of an arm prosthesis. Because there are relatively few primary arm amputees each year the expertise for their training has been centralized in a selected number of major centres or hospitals associated with those centres. A short period of training in one of these centres is strongly recommended as much can be learnt not only from the therapist in charge but also from the other amputees attending for training at the same time.

References

British Orthopaedic Association (1973) *Report of the Committee on Prosthetic and Orthopaedic Services in England, Wales and Northern Ireland.*

PART II

An Introduction to Arm Prosthetics

CHAPTER 7

History of Arm Prosthetics

Throughout the ages attempts have been made to fashion a replacement for the human arm that moves and looks natural. One of the earliest records is given by Pliny. In AD 61 he wrote that a Roman general, Marcus Sergius, had an iron hand made to hold his shield after losing his right hand in the Second Punic War (218–201 BC).

There are several records of artificial limbs in the early and middle sixteenth century. In particular Ambroise Paré, the great French military surgeon, describes artificial arms and legs which he claimed could be reproduced by any locksmith. These artificial arms had hands which, after being set in a position passively, were then locked by the other hand. He also designed cosmetic hands of moulded leather and paper which held such objects as a pen. Other records from the sixteenth century are of artificial arms which were jointed and therefore capable of passive movement at the elbow and wrist as well as the fingers. These prostheses seem to have been available only to the wealthy while the majority managed with a simple hook and leather socket fastened to the body with straps.

It was not until the early nineteenth century that further advances were made. After the Napoleonic Wars a Berlin dentist, Peter Baliff, appears to have been the first person to use the trunk and shoulder girdle muscles as sources of power to give grasp and release to the hand. He used the movement of the sound shoulder to open the artificial hand while a spring action kept it closed. Since it was designed only for a below-elbow amputee and had a very weak grasp it had little practical value. In 1844 a Dutch sculptor, Van Peeterssen, designed the first arm for the above-elbow amputee in which Baliff's principle was applied to bend the elbow.

Once again it was war that stimulated further advances in upper limb prosthetic design. In 1860, after the Crimean and Italian campaigns, the French were left with a large number of amputees. The

Comte de Beaufort fitted them with a shoulder harness to control an artificial arm. He developed a simple hand, with a movable thumb, and a more complicated one in which repeated pulls on the same cord opened and closed the fingers. He also invented an above-elbow prosthesis in which the elbow was controlled by pressure against a lever at the side of the chest. But perhaps the most important innovation was a double spring hook for holding objects, which was the forerunner of the modern split hook. This appliance did not seem to be very popular at the time, for writings by Gripouilleau and others describe that the practice in France was to construct simple appliances which fitted into the prosthesis and fastened on to a labourer's tools. Nor do there seem to have been further advances in the design of mechanical hands, which were looked on merely as something to 'raise a hat or carry a cane' (Wellerson 1958).

This trend continued until after the First World War, when a wide range of speciality tools was developed in Europe, while in North America split hooks were more favoured for general use. In recent years alternative styled split hooks have become available in Britain, to increase their value for a wide range of activities. Selective use of speciality tools has continued and can often make it easier for the arm amputee to compete in open industry and pursue his chosen hobbies.

The development of prostheses during the twentieth century has been in an increasing use of synthetic materials in the fabricating of sockets, prosthesis and harness (known as appendages in the United Kingdom). More recently there has been research into the use of external power to activate the prosthesis.

During the last thirty-five years the importance of training arm amputees to use their prostheses has had increasing recognition, with facilities now available for all arm amputees to receive training either at the local limb-fitting centre or in the occupational therapy department of a specified hospital within the area. At Bridge of Earn Hospital it was found that 9 out of 10 of those who had received training used their prostheses actively whereas only half (6 out of 12) of those who had no training did so (Carter et al. 1970). This was despite the fact that three-quarters of those who had no training were below-elbow amputees compared with half of those who had training; the remaining half of the trained group had lost their arm above the elbow. At Roehampton three surveys were carried out in 1961–6, 1969–72 and 1974–6. Questionnaires were sent to all single arm amputees who had completed their training between one and two years previously and had no additional disability. Of 367 questionnaires sent out 254 were returned, giving a 69% response. The surveys were designed to try to discover whether arm amputees wore and use their prostheses and for which activities they found them useful. The questionnaire was modified in format after the first series to ensure that the wording was not influencing the response, which was surprisingly consistent through the three surveys. It was found that 73% of those that replied wore their prostheses and less than 3% had discarded them. Just over half of the total used their prostheses actively at work with 48% using a split hook. A further 32% used a split hook at home with only 20% not using it at all. These results contrast with those of Dr Roman in his survey in Liverpool in 1967, when he found that out of a total of 316 only 11% used a split hook regularly, 21% used it occasionally and 67% had discarded it. The survey at Roehampton covered only those amputees who had recently completed training, whereas it is understood that Dr Roman's questionnaire was sent to all arm amputees within a fixed geographical area. The surveys are not therefore strictly comparable, but do seem to indicate that training influences the degree to which the prosthesis is used actively.

References

Carter, I., Torrance, W. N. & Merry, P. H. (1970) Functional results following amputation of the upper limb. *Artif. Limbs Appliances, 81,* 137–41.

Wellerson, T. L. (1958) *A Manual for Occupational Therapists on the Rehabilitation of Upper Extremity Amputees.* Dubuque, Iowa: Wm. C. Brown.

CHAPTER 8

Types of Prostheses

An amputee wants a prosthesis for one or both of two reasons: to improve his appearance and to increase his function. An arm prosthesis is therefore designed with one or both of these aims in mind.

Few people are satisfied with the present appearance of the most functional arm. The constraints imposed by trying to provide maximum function using the minimum of effort appear to be incompatible with an acceptable level of cosmesis. The majority of people are concerned with looking as normal as possible and so opt for the cosmetically acceptable but relatively non-functional prosthesis for use in public when increased function might make them look 'different'.

We therefore have three main groups of artificial arms:

1. Cosmetic, with no attempt to provide function.
2. Functional when the constraints of appearance are kept to the minimum so that maximum function can be achieved.
3. Functional and cosmetic when an attempt is made to provide both, often to their mutual detriment. The majority of prostheses supplied in the United Kingdom fall into this last group.

A prosthesis must have a rigid construction to give it shape and to provide fixed points for control systems. It can be endoskeletal or exoskeletal. The endoskeletal prosthesis has an internal rigid structure clad with whatever material is considered the most suitable for the purpose of the prosthesis, while an exoskeletal prosthesis has an external rigidity usually moulded to the shape required before completion. Until very recent years the majority of prostheses were of exoskeletal design. With the development of new materials, endoskeletal prostheses for both upper and lower limbs are beginning to find favour. Not only can they be of modular construction, so that production costs are kept to a minimum, but they can be more easily 'kept soft' to make them more cosmetically acceptable. A purely cosmetic prosthesis will probably be of endoskeletal design while functional or functional/cosmetic arm prostheses are more likely to be exoskeletal.

A cosmetic prosthesis will be held on to the body with the minimum of straps compatible with stability, while a prosthesis that aspires to any active function must have additional straps to harness the function of another part of the body to operate the prosthesis.

The most usual type of prostheses issued to a new arm amputee in the United Kingdom is a cable-controlled functional prosthesis. This is supplied with a detachable cosmetic hand for dress purposes and one or more working appliances. It will be of exoskeletal construction and made from a plastic material or leather or a combination of the two. It will have wrist and elbow units of light metal with metal knobs or levers controlling these movements.

These prostheses divide themselves into two main groups: those for amputations below the elbow and those for amputations above the elbow, with further subdivisions according to the level of amputation and the purpose for which they are to be used.

In the United Kingdom the prostheses for the various levels of amputations are identified by letters with a number to differentiate the weight or strength of the prosthesis. This is to ensure a consistent level of production and to try to eliminate misunderstanding about the type of prosthesis required (Table 1). Although this is mainly the concern of limb-fitting surgeons, prosthetists and technical officers, it is useful for others working with amputees to be familiar with the terminology. Although this system tends to standardize the prostheses available, it is possible to cater for individual requirements, and it is only occasionally that a 'special' prosthesis has to be sanctioned.

Table 1. Prostheses Available

Amputation	Heavy working: 1	Light working: 2	Dress: 3
Partially mutilated hand		Working	Cosmetic hand
Through-wrist	G1	Split-socket	Cosmetic hand
Long below-elbow	F1	F2	F3
Short below-elbow	E1	E2	E3
Through-elbow	D1	D2	D3
Above-elbow	B1	B2	B3
Through-shoulder	A1	A2	A3
Forequarter	—	Working	Cap only

Below-elbow prostheses

LONG BELOW-ELBOW

The below-elbow prosthesis consists of a forearm section, a wrist unit and a detachable hand, held in place by either a figure-of-eight appendage incorporating a control cable (Fig. 13) or a supracondylar cuff with a single loop harness for the control cable. This cable can be attached to either a lever on the hand to move the thumb or the movable part of a gripping appliance. If the prosthesis is to be purely cosmetic the figure-of-eight appendage or single loop harness may be unnecessary if the prosthesis can be held in place satisfactorily with a supracondylar cuff only. Below-elbow amputees, who have a figure-of-eight appendage with a control cable, can have these made detach-

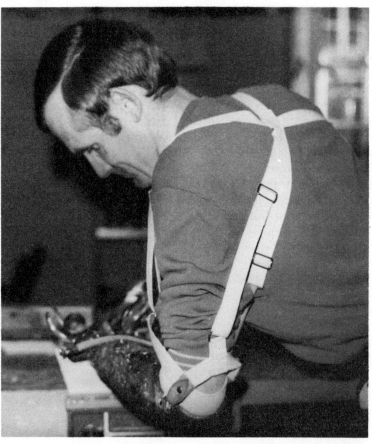

Fig. 13. The standard figure-of-eight appendage in general use on below-elbow prostheses in the United Kingdom.

able from the artificial limb so that it can be worn with a supracondylar cuff only on social occasions. Women, in particular, appreciate being able to do this as the straps across the back limit the style of clothes that they are able to wear. However, if the prosthesis is to be used for carrying heavy objects, with the elbow extended, the extra appendages may be necessary. Some below-elbow amputees have a stump suitable for a total contact socket of the Munster type, a German technique widely used for this type of fitting. This extends behind the olecranon to provide the necessary stability, and so prevents full elbow extension, but requires no straps for suspension. A single loop harness, similar to that used in conjunction with the supracondylar cuff, is the only appendage necessary to convert it into a working prosthesis.

The wrist unit allows the hand or appliance to be rotated through 360°. It is held by friction in any of 12 positions and can be locked in each of these by moving a small lever on the forearm to allow a pin to engage in a hole in the base plate of the hand or adaptor of the appliance. When this lever is pushed in the opposite direction the hand or appliance is released and pushed from the wrist unit by a spring action. This enables an amputee to release the catch before removing the hand or appliance from the forearm.

SHORT BELOW-ELBOW

When the stump is short a cup socket will usually be necessary to give a satisfactory prosthetic fit. This may be made of plastic or leather or a combination of the two. The forearm may be shortened to make the prosthesis easier to control. The wrist unit is then situated proximal to the natural wrist, allowing for a slimmer oval wrist to be incorporated into the cosmetic hand. An amputee with a very short below-elbow stump may need to have an above-elbow corset to keep the prosthesis firmly in place. The amputee with a very short below-elbow stump may also have difficulty in bringing the prosthetic arm up to the mouth owing to the limitation to elbow flexion caused by the prosthesis. For the single arm amputee this will not noticeably limit the function of the prosthesis but for a double arm amputee it can be crippling, especially if the other arm is amputated at the same level or higher. In these cases a step-up elbow joint should be fitted. The socket for the stump is separate from the forearm unit allowing a ratio of 2:1 movement of forearm unit to stump. A below-elbow amputee who has a weak or absent triceps muscle, as is often found after a brachial plexus lesion, may need an external hinge with a bolt lock between socket and above-elbow corset, so that he can stabilize his elbow while putting tension on the operating cord (see p. 45).

THROUGH-WRIST

Should a person with a through-wrist amputation wish to engage in heavy work it may be necessary for him to have a prosthesis similar to that for a long below-elbow amputee. It will probably have to be made so that the socket can be opened to allow room for the broader distal condyles of the radius and ulnar to be inserted into the socket. This is a clumsy prosthesis as it makes the arm longer than normal and also makes it impossible to continue to use the valuable forearm movement of pronation/supination. If it is at all possible a functional split socket should be fitted instead so that this movement can be utilized. In essence, the standard socket is split, the middle third removed and the two halves are joined by two straps secured with studs to allow full rotation of the forearm (Fig. 14). The split hook is usually incorporated into the distal working socket, so the whole socket can easily be removed and replaced with a cosmetic hand. The appendage for this functional prosthesis is the same as for a below-elbow prosthesis but the cosmetic hand should not require any appendages as the flaring of the epicondyles provides good anchorage. The main disadvantage of this type of prosthesis is the difficulty in getting a stable comfortable fit of the distal working socket. This socket tends to pivot when any lateral pressure is put on the working appliance and so must be flared and well padded to secure a comfortable fit.

PARTIALLY MUTILATED HANDS

Although there is a semi-standard type of working appliance designed for these injuries it rarely proves satisfactory. Much greater success is achieved if a functional appliance can be designed for the specific purposes required, making the maximum use of the remnant of the hand. The standard appliance is a leather socket moulded over the remaining body of the hand, leaving any fingers or thumb free. A castellated fitting can be incorporated into this so that various appliances can be used and a metal opposition post, if appropriate, can also be included. A wrist cuff attached to the socket with two leather chapes and D-rings, allowing free wrist movement, may be necessary to give a secure fixation.

A tailor-made functional appliance for a person with part of their hand remaining will probably prove more successful and with so many easily moulded synthetic materials available it is often possible for the occupational therapist to make up a temporary working appliance in her department, modifying it while the patient is using it until the most satisfactory solution is arrived at. This can then be used as a model for a more permanent appliance to be made by the prosthetist or technician. Some of the possible solutions are described and illustrated by Tomaszewska et al. (1974).

A cosmetic prosthesis made to complete the hand so that it looks as normal as possible is available. It is usually made so that the remaining digits are left uncovered for sensation.

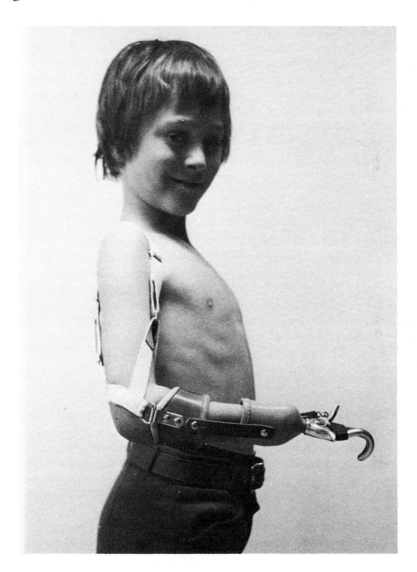

Fig. 14. A split socket for a through-wrist deficiency, allowing full rotation of the forearm.

Through-elbow prosthesis

As already mentioned in Chapter 2, a through-elbow amputation presents the prosthetist with the problem of marrying mechanical efficiency with appearance. The flared end formed by the epicondyles of the humerus often necessitates a socket that can be opened, with the associated cosmetic problem of straps or some alternative fastening. The prosthetic elbow hinges have to be external, which makes for a clumsy prosthesis and causes additional wear on clothes. A lateral mechanism cannot be incorporated into the prosthetic elbow and, although in theory it should be possible to cut down the socket to below the point of the shoulder and therefore cause less restriction to internal and external rotation, this is not always possible. The forearm, wrist unit and appendages are similar to that used for an above-elbow prosthesis.

Above-elbow prostheses

LONG ABOVE-ELBOW

The above-elbow prosthesis consists of an upper arm section moulded to fit over the stump and point of the shoulder, an elbow unit, forearm, wrist unit and detachable hand. The forearm can be full length or mid-forearm length. The whole is held in position by a three-point appendage which goes across the wearer's back and around the opposite shoulder. The elbow can be locked in seven positions including full extension. The movement to flex the elbow and to move the thumb or gripping appliance originates from a rounding of the shoulder girdle associated with flexion of the shoulder joint (Fig. 15).

To operate the locking mechanism of the elbow unit depression combined with extension at the glenohumeral joint is necessary. This is very much a trick movement, which is difficult to learn to use in conjunction with the abduction of the scapulae necessary to flex the elbow.

A valuable lateral friction movement is also incorporated in the standard elbow unit. This replaces the internal and external rotation of the shoulder, which is restricted by the socket and appendages, and allows the prosthetic forearm to be prepositioned into a convenient alignment in relation to the body, other hand, eye or mouth. There is a lock, similar to that on the wrist unit, for stabilizing this alignment in any one of five positions.

36

SHORT ABOVE–ELBOW

When the above-elbow stump is short a cup socket will be necessary and this may need to extend farther over the point of the shoulder to retain the prosthesis in the correct position. Because of the shorter length of lever available to move the prosthesis it is much more difficult for these amputees to get active full flexion of the elbow and to operate the elbow lock. Many of these patients will use a body swing movement to obtain the required degree of flexion and then operate the elbow lock manually.

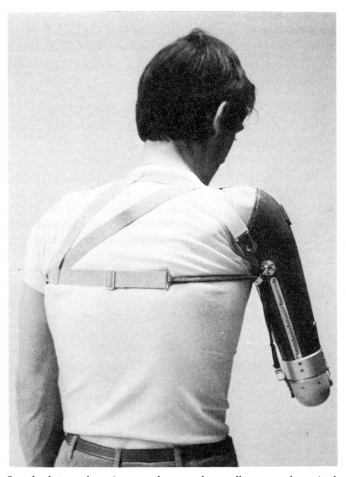

Fig. 15. Standard appendages in general use on above–elbow prostheses in the United Kingdom, with the operating cord under tension to flex the elbow.

THROUGH-SHOULDER

This prosthesis can have either a hinged or a rigid shoulder. Most amputees prefer the former as it allows a limited amount of free movement when the wearer changes position and so provides less of a drag on the body. It also makes dressing very much easier. Very few through-shoulder amputees can make much use of a cable-controlled prosthesis and unless there is a pressing need for functional grasp, when external power should be considered, they will find it less frustrating to concentrate on the use of the prosthesis in a passive, assistive role. However, most through-shoulder prostheses are fitted with an operating cable to the elbow. The prosthesis is made up of similar component parts to the above-elbow prosthesis, but either with the elbow lock strap riveted to the socket for manual operation or with a manual elbow lock knob on the forearm. The lock for the lateral movement is often omitted as unnecessary for the type of activities the wearer will be engaged in.

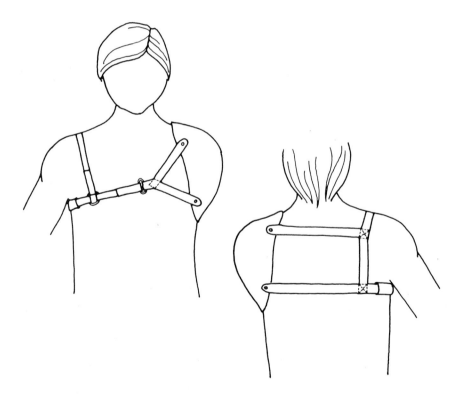

Fig. 16. The front and back views of the shoulder cap for a forequarter amputation.

FOREQUARTER

Once the clavicle and scapula are removed the shoulder assumes the curve of the rib cage so the prosthesis must provide a built-up shoulder cap on to which the artificial arm can be fixed. Because of the lack of bony protuberances and the pull of gravity it is very difficult to get a comfortable and secure fit without very tight straps around the body to hold the prosthesis in place. The wearer often finds this restricting and he may well choose to have a shoulder cap only and dispense with the arm part of the prosthesis. This will lessen the weight and therefore the tendency for the prosthesis to slip. The provision of a soft shoulder cap as soon as possible is beneficial. The psychological effect of wearing clothes that slip off the shoulder and advertise the loss in such an obvious way can intensify the natural depression of a person who has had to undergo such a disfiguring operation.

It is relatively easy to fabricate a soft shoulder cap from Plastazote lined with foam to fit comfortably over any necessary dressings, and this should be well within the capacity of any therapist familiar with handling these materials (Fig. 16). A sheet of 1 cm (0.5 in) Plastazote should be moulded over the amputated side of the thorax and trimmed to shape; roughly oval pieces of Plastazote, diminishing in size, are then bonded to the mould to bring the cap to nearly the same height and shape as the sound shoulder. The cap is then smoothed to get a good contour and a further sheet of 0.5–1.0 cm (0.25–0.5 in) Plastazote bonded over to give a good outline. Straps are then riveted on as indicated in Fig. 16, with a pull-back Velcro fastening in front. The strap should be partly of soft elastic to allow for a comfortable fit.

A more permanent shoulder cap can be provided later by the limb-fitting centre should the patient decide to continue with this form of prosthesis, or alternatively he can have a full arm prosthesis, which would have similar components to a prosthesis for a through-shoulder amputee.

Prostheses for double arm amputees

When two arm prostheses are fitted the appendages are normally linked together dispensing with the axilla loop. Some arm amputees like to have detachable appendages so that they can have a spare set fitting one prosthesis only. Blind double arm amputees are usually trained with one prosthesis only so that they have one stump free to feel with. They can then have a simple cosmetic prosthesis to wear on this arm for dress occasions.

References

Tomaszewska, J., Kapczyńska, A., Konieczna, D., Dembinska, J. & Miedzyblock, W. (1974) Solving individual problems with partial hand prostheses. *Interclin. Info. Bull.*, XIII (5), 7–13.

CHAPTER 9

Control and Sensory Feed-back

The types of controls on a functional prosthesis will depend on the level of amputation, whether one or two arms are involved and the degree of control and power that the amputee has in the remaining parts of his body.

In order to use a prosthesis it is necessary to have some knowledge of where the prosthesis is in space and its relationship to the object it is holding or about to pick up. When using one's own hand, and assuming an intact nervous system, this is provided along three complementary channels:

1. Touch sensation, giving information about the texture, weight and friction of the object touched or held.
2. Proprioception from muscle, joint and bone, giving an awareness of position in space.
3. Sight, identifying the position of the object to be touched or handled and giving information, based on experience, as to its size, density and surface.

When using a prosthesis channel 1 is absent and channel 2 is progressively impaired as the amputation becomes more proximal. This leaves only channel 3—sight—to help compensate for the lack of the other two. However, although an arm amputee is very dependent on vision for information of where his prosthesis is in space, he does get various clues from the friction and weight of his prosthesis and its appendages on his body. When the amputee lifts his arm the weight of the prosthesis is felt on the stump and the wearer soon learns by the degree and distribution of this weight the approximate angle of the prosthesis. Similarly the amputee receives sensory information from the tension of the straps and particularly of the operating cable, which tells him the degree of opening of the hand or other activated appliance and the degree of flexion of the forearm in the case of the above-elbow amputee.

When an external power source is provided this information from the control cable is removed and, because a much smaller and more delicate movement is required to open a valve or trigger a micro-switch, there is less feed-back of information from the controlling mechanism. Attempts to overcome this disadvantage of external power has led to the development of position servo systems, which can be incorporated into prostheses powered by both carbon dioxide and electricity. Other research has been into various types of anti-slip devices which are incorporated into the gripping surfaces of artificial hands. Some of these give off auditory signals while others are designed to give increasing pressure as slip starts to occur. These more sophisticated aids to sensory feed-back are still at the experimental stage and, although user trials have been started in some centres, they are not generally available. Certainly these more sophisticated sensory feed-back systems do seem to offer the possibility of improved function for the high-level amputee, but if they are to do so they must be sufficiently developed to give reliable performance with a low level of maintenance.

Control systems

In the United Kingdom external power is never routinely supplied if cable controls are considered to be satisfactory. Cable controls have been found to be more efficient overall than external power at its present level of development. Of all the advantages and disadvantages listed in Table 2, and others will no doubt have more to add, the questions of reliability and sensory feed-back are the lynch-pins in the choice. It is no good having a highly sophisticated prosthesis which spends even a quarter of its life needing repairs. The wearer no sooner learns to use it than he no longer has it and all the carefully established patterns of achievement are lost. The amputee then has either to change to a cable-controlled prosthesis and re-learn to use that or to manage without. Patterns of movement are not so easily learnt that one can shift naturally from one type of controls to another. It is not like driving a different car or even changing from car to boat or aeroplane. It is more like changing from riding a bicycle to operating a radio-controlled boat or aeroplane. It requires a different set of base skills, which have a long and often tedious apprenticeship.

Table 2. Control systems

Control system	Advantages	Disadvantages

Cable	Reliable
	Mechanically simple
	Few breakdowns
	Simple to replace or repair
	Easy to control
	Some feed-back of
	    proprioception
	Low cost
		May, be cosmetically
		    unacceptable
		Degree of function
		    dependent on available
		    body power
		Additional appendages
		    necessary

External power	Minimum movement or
	    muscle contracture
	    required to operate
	No cable to restrict
	    position in which
	    prosthesis is used
	Fewer external fittings,
	    giving a more stream-
	    lined appearance
	Minimum of harnessing
		Liability to breakdown
		Need for centralized
		    highly skilled technicians
		    and prosthetists to fit
		    and repair prosthesis
		Accommodation of power
		    source
		Noise of operation
		Little feed-back in
		    non-servo systems
		High cost

EXTERNAL POWER

The development of external power was given a stimulus by the thalidomide tragedy (1959–61) and by 1961 the first prosthesis powered by carbon dioxide was being fitted in Germany. In 1962 the first British child was fitted with a prosthesis made from parts imported from Germany. The design was then modified to suit British requirements and developments in the use of carbon dioxide as a power source continued at several centres in the United Kingdom. This type of control system has been found more suitable than cable controls for many limb-deficient children with complete absence of arms or very short phocomelia. Powered prostheses do, however, have several disadvantages and one should not conclude that all children with absent arms must have carbon dioxide powered prostheses. This will be discussed more fully in Chapter 15.

A carbon dioxide powered prosthesis is operated by valves which are opened and closed by small movements of any part of the body compatible with the function of the prosthesis. The most commonly used movements are those of the acromion processes (which are very prominent in most children with amelia or phocomelia), the phoco-melic digits, the stump within the socket or the trunk. Micro-switches can be controlled in a similar way or sometimes they are inserted within a cable system.

Electricity as a power source is also being used with increasing success. This can be used with either micro-switches or myoelectric controls. Early work done in the United Kingdom and Russia on myoelectric controls led to the fitting at Roehampton of an experimental arm prostheses with myoelectric controls in the early 1960s.

A myoelectric controlled prosthesis operates by harnessing the electrical potential produced by a contracting muscle to activate a battery-driven motor which, in turn, operates a prosthetic component (Trefler 1972). This can be a two-channel control system, as developed in Russia, which has a similar effect to that produced by a micro-switch, in that it has only an on/off control of the motor. An alternative system provides proportional control of the motor so that the stronger the myoelectric signal the greater the force or speed of movement.

Much of the present work on the use of micro-switches and EMG signals to control prostheses is being carried out in Canada and the United States of America. Work is also being done in Germany, Austria, Italy, Belgrade, Sweden and Japan, with particular emphasis on the development of electrically powered hands. In the United Kingdom research was originally carried out into both myoelectric and carbon dioxide powered prostheses, with resources eventually being concentrated on the development of prosthetic components using carbon dioxide as a power source. At the time it was felt that this would provide a quicker solution to a problem that would not wait on a research programme that might take a decade. Prostheses were needed within months. Research was carried out at four main clinical centres, three in England and one in Scotland, with additional work being done at non-clinical centres with special technical expertise. Originally it developed along two main lines. In England the emphasis was on providing power to individual joint movements, following the practice of Dr Marquadt in Heidelberg, while in Scotland Dr Simpson developed the idea of the linked wrist, elbow, shoulder movement which allows the hand/shoulder distance to be varied while main-taining the hand at a constant angle in relation to the horizontal. His practice has been to fit one highly functional prosthesis using control sites on both shoulders, whereas in England the tendency has been to try to fit two arm prostheses with complementary functions. More recent research at BRADU, Roehampton, has followed Dr Simpson's lead in producing the Radius Vector arm prosthesis. This has yet to be fitted with a position servo control system, which is an integral part of the Edinburgh or EPP (extended physiological proprioception) arm prosthesis.

Although research in the United Kingdom into carbon dioxide powered prostheses has been aimed at the needs of the congenital high-level bilateral arm deficiencies, some of the externally powered components can be usefully incorporated into conventional arm prostheses for the amputee with an additional problem (Chapters 14 and 18).

Despite the fact that much time, expertise and money have been devoted throughout the world to the development of external power for prostheses, they have not yet reached a degree of effectiveness and reliability equivalent to that of cable-operated prostheses. For this reason, if for no other, they are not at present fitted routinely in the United Kingdom to arm amputees who can make use of a cable-operated prosthesis.

CABLE CONTROL

The power used to operate a cable-controlled prosthesis is provided by the remaining muscles in the body. The movements most commonly used are those of the shoulder girdle, occasionally supplemented by those of the trunk and neck. Which specific movements are harnessed will depend on the level of amputation and the power and range of movement available. The principle of operating a cable-controlled prosthesis is to increase the distance between two fixed points on the body, therefore putting tension on a movable part of the prosthesis.

$$A --------- B --------- C$$

If the distance between B and C is increased there will be tension on A to move giving

$$A ---- B ------------- C$$

However, if A and B are fixed to two rigid structures with a pivot or joint between them the result is

It can therefore be seen that the greater the range of movement between B and C the greater the movement at the joint between A and B.

As the reverse movement is by either spring or gravity, power also becomes important. The greater the power of the body movement the stronger can be the spring or gripping action of the prosthesis, or the heavier the weight lifted against gravity.

This resistance can be varied by the position of the fixed point A in relation to the joint or pivot, for the nearer the pivot it is placed the greater the resistance but the smaller the movement needed to achieve a fixed degree of movement. However, it will be seen later that placing point A too far from the pivot (to reduce the power needed) can create other problems. To apply this principle to an arm prosthesis, tension is put on a cable to make the prosthetic elbow bend. This cable runs from the prosthetic forearm through a pulley on the upper arm, across the back, and into a loop around the opposite shoulder. When the back is rounded the distance between this loop and the pulley on the upper arm is increased, putting tension on the length of cable between the pulley and the prosthetic forearm and causing the elbow to flex (see Fig. 15). To operate a mechanical hand or appliance, the elbow joint must be made rigid so that the power can bypass this point and be exerted on the next movable joint in the hand or appliance. Tension on the cable will therefore cause the hand or appliance to open against a spring mechanism which normally keeps it closed. In a below-elbow prosthesis the cable will operate only on the hand or appliance if the elbow is maintained in the same position or slightly extended. The cable is normally routed on the front of the elbow, necessitating a good triceps muscle to counteract its pull.

References

Trefler, E. (1972) A comparison of control systems for upper extremity prosthetics. *Can. J. occup. Ther., 39* (2), 73–86.

CHAPTER 10

Temporary Prostheses

A successful user of an arm prosthesis must do more than just learn to control his prosthesis. He must establish patterns of movement which result in him using his prosthesis naturally in conjunction with his remaining arm. It must become habit to use the prosthesis for the majority of two-handed activities. To do this after a period, however brief, of being one-handed involves re-learning all those neurophysiological patterns of movement involving the use of two hands which are so slowly learnt in childhood. If, however, this period of one-handedness can be abolished or kept to a minimum of days, rather than weeks or months, learning will be limited to the techniques of using the prosthesis in conjunction with the other hand and the idea of using it in this way will feel natural.

A temporary prosthesis can be of two kinds. It can be either an immediate postoperative fitting (IPOF) or an early fitting. The application of a rigid dressing, which is an inherent part of the IPOF procedure, is said to be a sound surgical concept (Loughlin 1969), and is reported to improve the control of post-surgical oedema, reduce postoperative pain and speed up the conditioning of the stump. From the therapist's point of view it means that training in the use of the prosthesis can start immediately. Two-handed patterns of movement are not lost so re-learning, with reduced chances of success, is unnecessary. For the amputee it means an immediate reassurance of the continuing usefulness of his amputated arm, with a concurrent improvement in acceptance of amputation and a minimization of post-amputation shock and depression. In financial terms it should mean that the time between amputation and return to work is reduced. Many arm amputees can and do return to work with their temporary prosthesis.

For IPOF to be successfully carried out amputation and fabrication of the temporary prosthesis must be done by a skilled centralized team.

But most amputees lose their arms in accidents which may happen anywhere at any time and for this reason alone the opportunities to carry out this procedure have been limited. However, those reported (Loughlin 1969) do seem to indicate a higher rate of successful limb usage than any other procedure. This is supported by the six amputees treated by this method at Roehampton.

The next best alternative is the early fitting of a temporary prosthesis. If this can be carried out within days of amputation the success from the user angle is almost as good as from IPOF. The limbs can be made in a variety of ways but must fulfil the criteria of either speed of fabrication or adaptability of size to suit a variety of stumps. In North America (Bailey 1970; Reyburn 1971) and Australia (Wilson 1969) the most usual practice is to fabricate a plaster socket into which various prosthetic components may be incorporated; in the United Kingdom it is more likely that a new arm amputee will be supplied with a reconditioned prosthesis to use until his definitive limb can be made. A third method, which has been tried out successfully during the last few years at Roehampton with selected patients, is to fit the amputee with an adjustable socket for which he can be measured prior to amputation (see Fig. 17). This is worn over the stump bandage and can be adjusted to give firm and even pressure over the stump as the oedema disperses.

But since the majority of hospitals have neither the facilities nor the expertise to fit temporary prostheses it is vital that the amputee is referred to his nearest limb-fitting centre at the earliest possible moment. When an elective amputation is to be carried out this should be prior to amputation. In the more usual traumatic arm amputation it should be immediately afterwards. Unfortunately referral is often delayed until the wound has healed and the next stage of treatment is being considered. So because of the difficulties in achieving IPOF or an early fitting in a limb-fitting centre and the importance of use of the amputated arm to the eventual acceptance and use of the prosthesis, every occupational and physiotherapist should be aware of the alternatives of adjustable gauntlets and plaster sockets.

The making and fitting of gauntlets has already been described (Chapter 4) and is well within the capabilities of any occupational therapist, physiotherapist or nurse who has the materials available. The making of a plaster socket requires some experience of stump bandaging as these principles are used when applying the plaster bandage. A tubular stockinette mitt is first made to fit snugly over the stump, with any necessary stitching positioned on the lateral aspect of the stump and avoiding any tender areas. Lengths of 7 cm (3 in) plaster bandage are then placed over the end of the stump as for turns 1, 2 and 3 of stump bandaging, followed by further lengths of plaster bandage in overlapping figures-of-eight to give an even pressure on the stump. While making the socket the below-elbow stump should be held in a neutral mid-position, between pronation and supination, and be free to flex at the elbow. The above-elbow stump should be slightly abducted and flexed approximately 10° and care should be taken to extend the rear wing of the socket sufficiently to prevent rotation on the stump and to cut it away sufficiently on the top and front to allow free abduction and forward flexion. As Reyburn says, a plaster socket, held in position with a figure-of-eight appendage, is often more satisfactory than an elastic stump bandage for an above-elbow amputee. It can be fitted before the stump is ready for a temporary prosthesis and because it is secure the amputee can be encouraged to exercise his stump in a more active manner than when wearing only an elastic bandage. However, the aim is to fit a useful extension to this plaster socket, as described by Wilson (1969), Loughlin (1969), Bailey (1970) and Reyburn (1971). Therapists unfamiliar with the fitting and training of arm amputees would be well advised to limit their fitting to a simple extension to the plaster socket. More sophisticated prostheses place additional strains on the stump which may not have been allowed for in the initial fabrication of the socket. This prosthetic extension should be designed to equalize length and to allow the amputee to use his temporary prosthesis in a passive helping role in bimanual activities. Simple lightweight devices are usually easier to control and therefore more likely to be used by a patient in the early days after amputation when the stump is still tender.

Each year a few patients undergo amputation due to disease. These elective amputations are the ones that lend themselves to IPOF procedures or the fitting of adjustable pre-made prostheses. Both have been carried out on a limited number of patients at Roehampton with the latter being in current favour. They have all been above-elbow amputees and have started their training within one to four days after amputation.

The adjustable prosthesis is made with conventional elbow and forearm units and moulded leather upper arm split in the front. This is fastened with Velcro straps which completely surround the upper arm and so allow for infinite adjustment (Fig. 17). The prosthesis is worn over either an elastic bandage, put on in the conventional way but fastened with adhesive tape rather than a pin, or a Plastazote lining socket. This ensures an even firm pressure as well as protection to the stump in the immediate postoperative period. A programme geared to whole-day wearing should be started and achieved by the end of the first week. Training activities should be graded, initially with periods of passive use in bimanual activities and short supervised periods of specific prosthetic training, gradually changing to longer periods spent on specific prosthetic training activities. Such is the keenness of amputees trained in this way that care must be taken not to let them overstress their stumps.

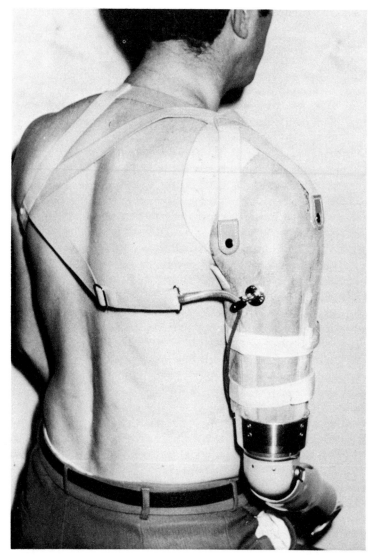

Fig. 17. An adjustable temporary prosthesis for immediate postoperative fitting of an above-elbow amputee.

References

Loughlin, E., Stanford, J. W. & Phelps, M. (1969) Immediate post-surgical fitting of a bilateral below-elbow amputee. A report. *Prosthetics Int., 3(8)*, 47–9.

Bailey, R. B. (1970) An upper extremity prosthetic training arm. *Am. J. occup. Ther., xxiv(5)*, 357–9.

Reyburn, T. V. (1971) A method of early prosthetic training for upper extremity amputees. *Artif. Limbs, 15(2)*, 1–5.

Wilson, E. B. (1969) Pre-prosthetic training for the upper extremity amputee. *Br. J. occup. Ther., 32(11)*, 17–21.

CHAPTER 11

Terminal Devices

Most arm amputees find that the standard hand issued in the United Kingdom has very limited function. The more sophisticated mechanical hand are not readily available under the National Health Service to single arm amputees and if the amputee wishes to use his prosthesis for more than simple steadying and supporting he will need an alternative appliance. The one most commonly used throughout the world is the split hook. Various designs are available, depending on the purpose for which it will be used. Most split hooks are designed with one fixed and one movable jaw and are kept closed with springs or rubber bands. The amputee exerts force to open these and relaxes to allow them to close. Although this is the opposite to the physiological functioning of the hand it does allow the amputee to 'forget' the act of holding an object once it has been grasped and concentrate on the activity itself.

Split hooks

The hook-shape split hook (Steeper's spring-loaded or rubber-covered) has been now largely superseded by the canted split hook (Dorrance or Steeper adult) because of its greater precision and flexibility (Fig. 18). All new amputees will be routinely supplied with this type of split hook unless a special request for the older type is made. Hook-shape split hooks are still available for those familiar in their use who do not wish to change.

The canted split hook is available in either steel or duralumin. It has parallel opening to a maximum of 10 cm (4.25 in) with a non-slip material bonded to the gripping surfaces, except for the tips which are of serrated metal to give a precision grip. One jaw is curved to facilitate carrying and to allow for a three-point grasp using the operating lever for support. The hook is kept closed by flexible rubber bands which can be easily graded from light to strong by adding extra bands.

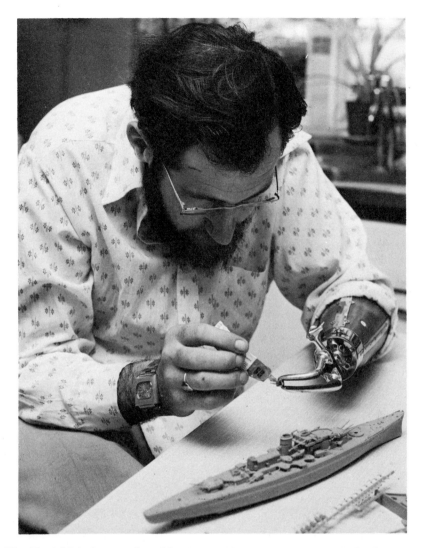

Fig. 18. A high degree of precision is possible with this canted split hook.

Successful use of the split hook depends mainly on practice. Unfortunately some people are put off from persevering with this tool because of its appearance and the connotations attached to the idea of a hook. Often their first attempts to use a split hook are not very successful because they do not know how to use it to exploit its full potential. Certain basic rules must be remembered in the early stages of training if the amputee is not to become discouraged in learning to use the split hook.

1. When picking up an object the rigid finger should be placed next to the object so that the movable finger closes on to it without knocking the object over.

2. The split hook should be pre-positioned by rotating it in the prosthetic forearm so that it can be aligned with the object to be picked up or used.

3. The above-elbow amputee also needs to pre-position both the degree of elbow flexion and the position of the lateral.

4. The height of the working surface is important and ideally should be below the level of the elbow when the arm is relaxed. Most new arm amputees find it easier to work standing or sitting on a high stool.

5. It is impossible to pick up and hold an object that requires a greater strength of grasp than is given by the tension of the rubber bands or springs holding the split hook closed, by relying on grasp only. To overcome this the rigid jaw of the split hook should be positioned underneath the object to support it, so that a less powerful grip is required, e.g. when carrying a plate or tray.

6. The shape of the split hook can also be exploited for pulling and carrying by using the hook of the fingers.

7. When holding a tool or an object on which pressure is to be exerted it must be positioned in the split hook so as to give a three point grip with the force transmitted against a rigid part of the split hook, e.g. holding a knife, spanner or pencil (see Fig. 29).

Alternative appliances

Once the control and use of the split hook has been mastered the arm amputee should try other appliances and decide for himself whether they would help him to pursue work and hobby interests.

There is a wide selection of standard appliances available in the United Kingdom and it is also possible for special appliances to be tailor-made. Some of the standard appliances are versatile and others are designed for specific activities. It is easy to think, in the early days of wearing a prosthesis, that a different appliance for each job would be useful. However, experienced arm amputees use a minimum of appliances. The nuisance of having to change appliances and carry alternative appliances around encourages versatile use of one or possibly two for all types of activity.

Alternative appliances fall into two groups: static and active. Static appliances do not require the operating cord and are in the form of a specialist tool for holding down objects or for attaching to a tool. Active appliances have the ability to grasp and provide active prehension like the split hook once the operating cord is attached. They differ only from the split hook in shape and type of gripping surface. Some of these active appliances have positive opening and some positive closing. The positive closing appliances have a locking mechanism so that tension on the operating cord does not need to be maintained to retain grasp. Most of these appliances can be used without an operating cord. This is useful for the high level amputee who cannot operate a split hook with a good grasp and yet may want to be able to hold an object firmly.

Although few alternative appliances are now issued, occasionally one will assist in the achievement of a skill. No appliance should be issued without the amputee having had the opportunity to try it out. Frequently it is not an alternative tool that is required but more practice in using the split hook.

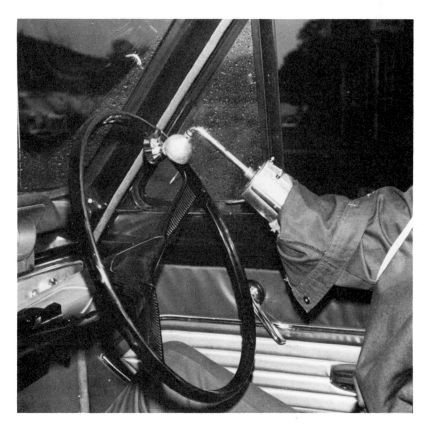

Fig. 19. Positive control of the steering wheel, coupled with quick release, are features of the driving cup and ball.

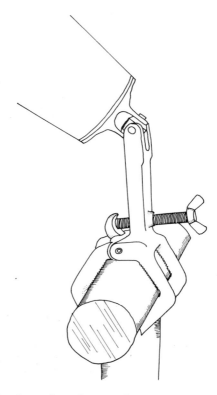

Fig. 20. A spade grip clamped on the top of a spade handle.

DRIVING CUP AND BALL

The ball is attached to the steering wheel (Fig. 19) and the cup either has a stem which fits into the wrist unit or screws into the palm of the hand. The cup fits over the ball, giving positive control of the wheel and yet is easy to remove in an emergency. The cup will also fit over the top of most standard gear levers, enabling a below-elbow amputee to change gear if the amputation is on the corresponding side. Recent arm amputees are advised to start with the separate cup appliance, rather than the cup screwed into the palm of the hand, as the hand can obscure the cup and make precise placement of the cup on the ball difficult.

SPADE GRIP

A useful appliance for anyone doing a lot of digging or shovelling or for playing games such as cricket. It is clamped on to the tool and,

56

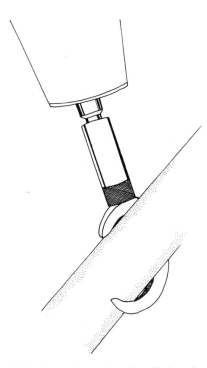

Fig. 21. The William C hook used on a long-handled tool.

having a universal joint, allows the other hand to control the tool using the spade grip as a pivot point (Fig. 20). It can also be used on shears, hoes, rakes, brooms, wheelbarrows, etc. It is a useful tool for the gardener but, because it has to be clamped on to the tool with the other hand and tends to damage the handles of the tools, it is not always popular. If used frequently on several tools it is possible to have more than one so that they can be left in situ.

WILLIAM C HOOK

A C-shaped hook with a strong spring in the shaft enabling it to have a two-point grip of a tool handle by stump pressure (Fig. 21). A very useful tool for the below-elbow amputee engaged in heavy outdoor work. It is versatile, has a smooth, shiny surface and so will not damage sacks, wood, etc. It is a difficult tool to learn to use as it requires considerable power in the stump, often more than the amputee has when receiving his initial training.

ANDERSON AND WHITELAW (A & W) TOOLHOLDER

This is a useful clamp for round-handled tools such as chisels. It takes both large and small diameters and is designed so that the tool can be set at various angles.

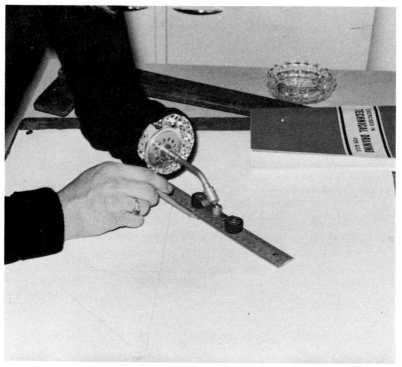

Fig. 22. The combined office and typing appliance is a simple, lightweight tool for a draftsman or office worker.

COMBINED OFFICE AND TYPING APPLIANCE

This is good for both typing and holding a ruler steady (Fig. 22). A typing peg and the two-pronged office appliance are also available but more limited in use.

PLIERS

These are available in three types, which are all positive closing and have either a locking screw or a lever to maintain the grasp. One of these tools is sometimes favoured by mechanics when ordinary pliers would be necessary.

PART III

The Adult Arm Amputee

CHAPTER 12

Learning to Live with One Artificial Arm

Psychological effect of losing a hand

How many of us have ever considered what it would be like to lose a hand? It is not a pleasant thought and most people have no reason to think that it will happen to them. But it does happen to some people each year: in 1974 at least 280 people lost an arm in England, none of whom could have expected such a thing to happen. Because it is not only an uncommon accident but also a mutilating one, the staff of hospitals are shocked as well as the patients. One might expect hospital staff to be used to seeing a limb amputated. In England in 1974 over 5000 people lost one or both legs; but the loss of a leg can be hidden. The patient sits in bed or a chair swathed in a blanket below the waist. The loss of an arm cannot be hidden either consciously or unconsciously from either staff or patient. The staff can walk away but the amputee can only raise his eyes from where his hand should be to escape the reminder that it has gone for ever. Most amputees appear remarkably stoical about their loss immediately after the accident, but what hidden turmoil there must be!

If we have been born with two functional hands we use them to complement each other. Suddenly the amputee finds himself with only one and he is at a loss to know how to do many simple everyday activities such as tying his shoelaces and fastening the top of his trousers. A woman finds she cannot fasten her bra or take the top off her lipstick. How does one cut up one's meat or open a door with both a Yale lock and a handle? There are hundreds of activities for which we normally use two hands automatically and which suddenly become a problem. These are the practical problems of losing a hand, which are relatively simple to solve. But what about the psychological problems? How does the amputee see himself after this very mutilating accident or operation? How is his loss going to effect how he thinks of himself in relation to others? Will he feel incomplete, an object of pity to his family and friends? He knows how he thought of other handicapped people. Now he is the handicapped person. Dr Fishman (1959) writes in his article on 'Amputee Needs, Frustrations and Behaviour' that the amputee finds seven of his basic needs frustrated to some extent by his amputation. These needs are physical function, cosmesis, comfort, energy cost, achievement, economic security and respect and status. This book concerns itself with all these aspects, with the object of helping the amputee achieve his full potential.

Before we, the able-bodied with two hands, can help the person who has lost a hand we must examine how we feel about amputation, recognizing it as a mutilation of the body and as such possibly repulsive. Can we look at and handle the remnant of a limb without feeling squeamish and treat the situation as a perfectly ordinary occurrence? Unless we can, our relationship with the amputee will be affected and because of this we will be less able to help him adjust to his loss. Many people cover up how they truly feel by being brusque and matter-of-fact, but this can make them appear unfeeling and unsympathetic. Yet sympathy and interest in a person's problems are essential to a good working relationship between staff and patients. Interest in their problems implies having time to listen and this is another way that help can be given to the amputee. In industry mechanization is less productive if consideration is not given to the people who work the machinery. Likewise with amputees, time needs to be spent listening to the patient in order to evaluate his needs before deciding what one can offer in the way of help. Fewer prostheses and appliances would rust in cupboards if more time were spent in discovering the best equipment to suit a person's needs, rather than issuing them routinely with standardized equipment according to sex, physique and occupation. If we know what is available we can be selective in the help offered to the new amputee.

Counselling is very important at this stage. The amputee needs information on the practical aspects of arm wearing and use as well as help in coming to terms with his own feelings. The timing is important, as is the choice of councillor. This should usually be a professional person with some knowledge of the problems. Sometimes it can be helpful to meet another arm amputee, but it must be someone who has adjusted to his loss and is not still struggling with his own feelings of grief and rejection.

Training programme

The amputee must first learn how to put on his prosthesis and then how to control it. Subsequent training consists of three stages which, although overlapping, have specific aims. Throughout the training the therapist/patient role changes and matures from dependence to independence. The aims are as follows:

1. To learn control.
2. To use the prosthesis in bimanual activities.
3. To apply these skills in a natural and automatic manner to those work and hobby activities of interest and importance to that person.

The first stage is largely directed by the therapist, the second guided by her and for the third her role gradually changes to that of adviser or consultant, with the emphasis on the amputee working out the best method and choice of tool for himself. Active use of the prosthesis gradually becomes automatic. The amputee wishes to use his prosthesis rather than its use being imposed from outside.

In the first stage, control of the prosthesis is best taught along with cable control. It is much easier for the amputee to learn this control using a split hook rather than a hand. Even if he is adamant that he does not wish to use one outside the department, he should be told firmly that it will be easier for him to learn to control and use his prosthesis with a split hook, and that later he can decide for himself which terminal device he uses.

PUTTING ON AND TAKING OFF THE PROSTHESIS

One of the first things that an amputee should learn is how to put on and take off his own prosthesis, even if at first he is unable to do so completely independently. For the majority of single arm amputees this should present no problem. Difficulty should only occur when there is a severe additional disability.

The prosthesis should be worn over a vest or T-shirt with a cotton or woollen sock covering the stump. This is to prevent abrasions to the skin from friction from the prosthesis or appendages. The established limb wearer may be able to tolerate the appendages next to the skin, once it has hardened in the areas of friction, but he should not discard the stump sock for this also absorbs the perspiration of the stump which cannot evaporate naturally. Stump socks should be of natural fibres, rather than synthetic, except for those with a congenital absence who can often tolerate nylon stump socks. Stump socks are issued free of charge to all amputees in the United Kingdom and are available at the limb-fitting centre.

The method of putting on a prosthesis depends on the level of amputation.

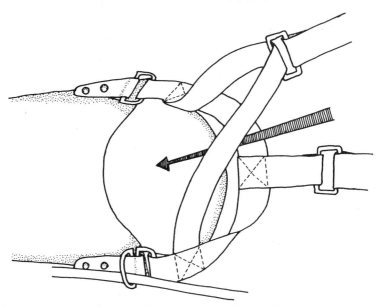

Fig. 23. Inserting a right below-elbow stump into the prosthesis.

Below-elbow

The stump should be inserted into the socket, passing in front of the appendages and under the V-strap which lies in front of the elbow (Fig. 23). The amputated arm should then be raised high enough for the appendages to hang free and the arm loop to be located. The sound arm is then taken behind the back and put through this loop. The shoulder straps can then be shrugged on to the shoulders: the procedure is very like putting on a coat. When taking off the prosthesis the shoulder strap on the amputated side is pushed back and off the shoulder, then the strap over the shoulder of the sound arm is pushed back, allowing that arm to be withdrawn from the shoulder loop of the appendage. The buckle on the shoulder loop should *not* be unfastened. The sound hand can then grasp the prosthesis and remove it from the stump. Putting on and taking off a total contact socket tends to vary from patient to patient and should be taught to the amputee by the prosthetist when he fits the prosthesis.

Above-elbow

An above-elbow prosthesis can be put on in one of three ways. For all of them it is easier if the elbow is locked at 90° flexion so that the operating cable is slack.

1. The shoulder loop is buckled to the loosest hole or if necessary an extension strap is added to give a larger loop. The stump is then pushed well into the socket, in front of any appendages, until the top of the socket rests over the point of the shoulder. The prosthesis is then raised and the trunk is side flexed towards the sound arm so that the appendages hang across the amputee's back. He can then insert his sound arm into the shoulder loop and shrug this on to this shoulder. The shoulder loop is then tightened to give a firm but comfortable fit and the elbow unlocked to check that full extension is possible.

2. For the second method the shoulder loop is unbuckled. Once the socket is firmly on the stump, the front strap of the shoulder loop is grasped in the sound hand and taken behind the head and over the shoulder of the sound arm. This can then be held under the chin or in the teeth while the buckle end of the shoulder loop is brought under the sound arm for fastening in front of the shoulder. If the prosthesis is inclined to slip off the stump during this procedure the amputee should sit or stand by a table or chest of a suitable height so that he can rest the prosthetic elbow and forearm on this.

3. The third method is only suitable for those amputees with a very short above-elbow stump. The shoulder loop is buckled in its normal position or looser and the sound arm inserted through it. The prosthesis is then grasped by the forearm and taken over and behind the head to rest on the amputated shoulder after the stump has been slipped into the socket. The strap and buckle can then be adjusted if necessary.

Through-shoulder

Usually method 3 described above for a short above-elbow stump is satisfactory. Sometimes a chest strap is fitted to give greater stability to the prosthesis and this is fastened once the prosthesis is in position.

Forequarter

These prostheses usually have to be put on by resting the prosthetic elbow and forearm (locked in 90° flexion) on a table, as described in method 2 for the above-elbow amputee, while fastening the straps around the body on opposite axilla. Occasionally such an amputee finds it easier to fasten his prosthesis initially while lying on his back on a bed. The straps can then be adjusted when sitting to get a comfortable fit.

Once the method of putting on and taking off the prosthesis is mastered the amputee must learn how to dress the prosthesis (p. 82), for sometimes it is easier to do this before putting on the prosthesis rather than after.

CONTROL OF THE SPLIT HOOK

The majority of split hooks in use today are of the voluntary opening variety and the operating mechanisms are described in Chapter 11.

It is better to start training with a fairly weak tension and restrict activities so that they can be successfully achieved with this tension, i.e. use light medium-sized objects with a high friction surface and avoid very small objects and those with a shiny or smooth surface. Having only a weak tension to pull against in the early stages will prevent fatigue, irritation of tender skin which has yet to be hardened to wearing a prosthesis and pressure on sensitive areas of the stump. Tension on the hook closure can be gradually built up during training so that by completion a realistic grasp is possible. It is difficult to be specific because age, sex, physique, level of amputation and length of time since amputation all influence the decision about the desirable tension. However, it is better to start cautiously with a half or single flat band on the first day, upgrading by half-bands each day to three to five bands providing no adverse symptoms are encountered.

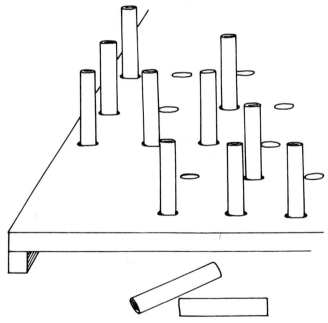

Fig. 24. A peg Solitaire board.

Grasp and release activities should be started with solid objects which are easy to hold in the split hook and will not 'slip away' when being grasped. A Solitaire or draught board with inset pegs (Fig. 24) or cotton reels on sticks (Fig. 25) are ideal as they give frequent repetition within a fairly restricted area, making adjustment of body position unnecessary. Games provide the best medium at this stage of the training and any board game, from snakes and ladders to chess, can be adapted to give repeated practice in grasp and release. Progression towards skilled use of the split hook can be made by varying:

1. The size and shape of counters (tall with parallel gripping surfaces progressing to short with curves).
2. The density of the counters (solid to soft foam).
3. The level of the board in relation to the player (with the optimum position being when the split hook is in front between hip and waist level).
4. The stability of the counters (light to heavy; inset or slotted to free-standing; flat-based to domed-based).

The amputee should also be encouraged to experiment in picking up various shaped and sized objects so that he begins to learn both the limitations and the potential of his split hook. Later this will be helpful to him when deciding when a split hook will be satisfactory and when an alternative appliance is needed.

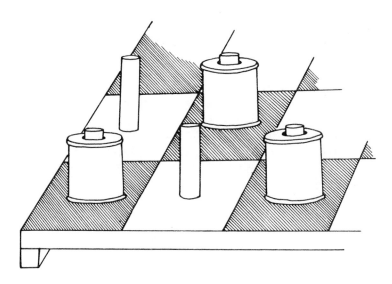

Fig. 25. Draughts, using cotton-reels on sticks.

PROPRIOCEPTION

As well as learning cable control the amputee is also learning to control his prosthesis in space. Additional training in this area can be given in a variety of ways without using grasp and release. It is important to avoid fatigue by interspersing specific cable-control activities with more general activities chosen to improve control of the prosthesis. Typing (p. 76) is an excellent activity for this purpose as the use of the prosthesis can be graded from space bar only to, eventually, half of the letters. Many simple bimanual activities can also be graded to demand the appropriate amount of precision in the use of the prosthesis. Activities such as holding papers steady for stamping or stapling, using a ruler, assembling files, steadying wood for sawing or material for cutting are suitable. Already the amputee is starting on the next stage of using the prosthesis to assist the other hand.

LEARNING ELBOW CONTROL

Once the arm amputee has learnt to control and use his split hook he should learn to control the elbow and elbow lock. With the single cable prostheses most commonly fitted, it is not possible to activate the split hook without first locking the elbow.

The elbow lock is a repeat pull mechanism which means that the same movement both locks and unlocks the elbow. The strap to operate the elbow lock is positioned at the front of the shoulder, stretching from the front of the elbow unit to a point just medial of the acromion process (Fig. 26). Tension has to be placed on this strap to move a lever at the front of the elbow unit. To obtain this tension the amputee must extend and slightly abduct his upper arm and at the same time depress it within the glenoid cavity (nudging a neighbour in the ribs is the nearest comparison). Most above-elbow amputees find this movement difficult to master as they either tend to extend the arm without pushing down or, if they do push down, tilt the whole body to that side rather than just pushing the arm down. They also tend to look down at the elbow-lock lever, rotating their trunk and increasing the difficulty of performing the elbow locking movement correctly.

It is therefore suggested that the above-elbow amputee should initially practise operating the elbow lock in front of a full length mirror, so that he can watch not only the elbow lock lever but also the level of his shoulders and the angle at which he holds his amputated arm. It is often easiest for him to learn the correct movement if the therapist can stand behind the amputated arm. She is then able to guide the upper arm passively in the correct sequence of movements, allowing the mechanism to lock and unlock while supporting the forearm so that no extra weight is placed on the elbow mechanism.

Because the mechanism is of a repeat pull type it is essential that the lever drops to the bottom of the slot before tension is placed on it, otherwise the mechanics of this type of lock do not work. It is therefore advisable that the amputee is taught initially to bring his prosthetic arm forward and across the body before attempting to extend backwards to unlock or lock the joint. This makes the sequence of movements to either lock or unlock the elbow joint as follows:

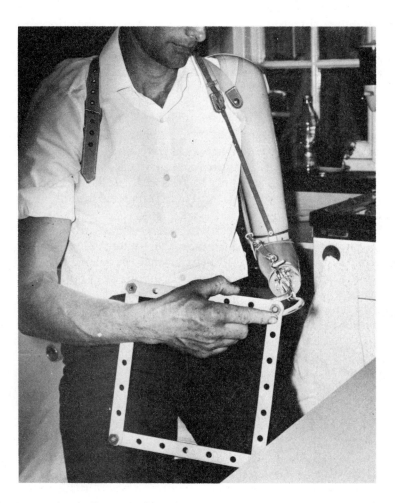

Fig. 26. An above-elbow prosthesis showing the position of the elbow-locking strap, and the prosthesis being used for a bimanual training activity.

69

1. Forward flex to allow lever to drop to bottom of slot.
2. Extend and slightly abduct the arm, pushing the elbow down towards the floor without altering the level of shoulders or trunk position.

Once this sequence of movements has been mastered, first with the therapist holding the prosthetic forearm and then with the amputee holding it himself, control of the forearm position while unlocking the elbow and later locking it must be learnt. To unlock the elbow without the forearm supported, slight tension must be placed on the operating cord to raise the weight of the forearm from the locking mechanism. The amputee therefore has to learn to maintain a position of slight scapula abduction while operating the elbow lock mechanism. Once the lock is released he can relax and allow the forearm to extend by pull of gravity. Finally he has to learn to flex the elbow and hold it in the desired position while locking the elbow.

Obviously all this is going to take several days to master and must be taken step by step within the amputee's physical and mental capacity. But once this last stage has been reached it is possible to devise games and activities which necessitate locking and unlocking the elbow at different levels. A ladder scoreboard used in conjunction with any scoring game is an easy way to achieve this. Placing objects to be used in an assembly job on different height shelves is another means of achieving the same end.

Most above-elbow amputees who master the control of the elbow lock, discover that they can shorten the routine when moving the forearm from one locked position to another. By raising the lock lever only partially the elbow movement becomes free but returns into lock as soon as the tension is removed from the lever.

Many single arm amputees never learn shoulder control of the elbow lock because they have not had enough tuition and practice. It is too easy to reach across and pull the lock strap with the other hand. Without shoulder control the above-elbow amputee will always be at a disadvantage when doing bimanual activities. There is no reason why the majority of above-elbow amputees cannot learn this control. One never finds a bilateral arm amputee unable to control his elbow lock by shoulder movements: he has to, for he has no hand to reach across with.

USING THE PROSTHESIS FOR BIMANUAL ACTIVITIES

To train an amputee to make the maximum use of the prosthesis an activity should be used that demands the use of the prosthesis as well as the other hand, and is also enjoyed by the patient. Some activities lend themselves to graded use of the prosthesis and it is easy to fall into the routine of using these when with a little extra thought and imagination more enjoyable activity could be adapted to give the same end result.

During the initial phase of training it should be possible to study the patient to discover what type of activity will interest him. Even so there are limits set by the prosthesis and the degree of control learnt at a particular stage. Although it is physically easier for the amputee to start bimanual activities with a split hook and then progress to using other tools or a hand, occasionally this process has to be reversed because of the attitude of the patient to his amputation and/or the wearing of a split hook. When amputees are treated as groups this is less of a problem as the new amputee quickly sees the practical advantages of the split hook over the hand for most activities.

By this stage the amputee should be reasonably familiar with the operation of the split hook but he will not yet have fully grasped its potential or its limitations. A little time should be spent in

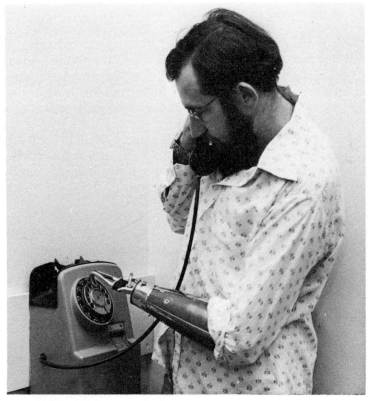

Fig. 27. Using a split hook to dial on the telephone.

71

demonstrating the features of the split hook and explaining how these can be used to help the amputee to pick up and hold objects of various sizes, shapes and density (Chapter 11). It is important to explain to him that force can be transmitted from the stump down through the rigid jaw of the split hook and that the hook can be turned through 360° and locked in position if necessary. This not only affects the line-up of the opening of the split hook but also enables the amputee to use this rigidity and force to give stability and power to the prosthesis. The operation of the elbow lock and lateral mechanism (p. 36) should also be demonstrated, although the shoulder control of the elbow-locking mechanism may not yet have been taught. The amputee should be shown the knob that locks and unlocks the lateral and it should be explained to him that keeping it unlocked in the early stages of training and when engaged in strenuous activities acts as a protection to his stump. Any undue strain will be absorbed by the friction action of the lateral rather than his newly amputated and perhaps tender stump.

Suitable activities within the scope of the average occupational therapy department could include woodwork, metalwork, light assembly work, weaving, technical drawing, typing, clerical work, gardening, sewing, knitting, cooking, washing up, billiards, cricket and table tennis. Other incidental activities, such as using a telephone (Fig. 27), making tea and coffee for the other patients and carrying it around on a tray or helping to move boxes and furniture, should be encouraged, as they foster the natural use of the prosthesis for every-day activities.

Let us look at some of these activities in more detail to see how they can be used for training in the use of the prosthesis and how they are most easily achieved as an on-going activity. Although the prosthesis normally plays the assistive role in bimanual activities there can be exceptions, either when the dominant hand has been lost or when the assisting hand would normally be required to have a greater degree of manual dexterity than the dominant one. Safety is another factor that should influence how some skills are carried out. As a general principle single arm amputees should be encouraged to use all sharp or danger-ous tools in their own hand. Not only will they have greater control of the tool, but should the tool slip only the prosthesis will be damaged and *not* their only hand.

Woodwork

Woodwork is one of the best media for training a single arm amputee. It demands the use of the prosthesis to help the sound hand in most of its processes, can easily be graded in degree of skill required and has a satisfying end product. For most of the processes the prosthesis will play the assistive role.

1. Sawing and hammering should be done with the sound arm in the interests of safety, regardless of original dominance. The rare exception is when a skilled craftsman is not able to reach a sufficiently high standard by this method.

2. Holding the wood on a bench hook for sawing should be encouraged as it increases the power of triceps.

3. When putting wood in a vice the wood should either be held in the split hook and fixed with the other hand or *vice versa*. Final tightening will usually have to be done with the sound hand.

4. When sawing the split hook is used as a guide for the saw much as one would use the back of the thumb.

5. When planing place the split hook on the forward knob of the plane. Some amputees prefer to turn the split hook so that the points face upwards (Fig. 28); above-elbow amputees often find it easier to

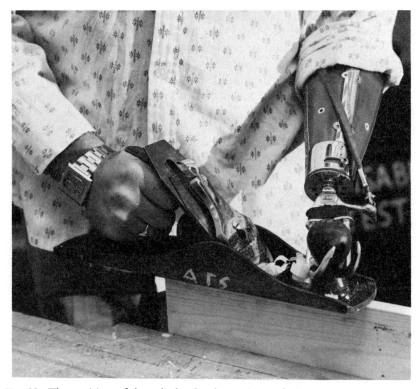

Fig. 28. The position of the split hook when using a plane.

have a free elbow and lateral and some like to disconnect the operating cable to the split hook as this can restrict shoulder movement or cause the split hook to open unintentionally; this sometimes occurs in the early stages when the tension against which the amputee is able to open the split hook is still not very great.

6. Sanding can be made into a bimanual activity by using a long sanding block with two cotton reels on top for grasp.

7. When using a hand drill the amputee should hold the side handle with his split hook turned 90°, so that the rigid jaw of the hook is on top, and turn the handle with the sound hand. A few below-elbow amputees who can manage a hook with a good grip will be able to hold the top handle and occasionally a below-elbow amputee will opt to turn the handle with his prosthesis. There is no correct way: the one chosen should be the one which is easiest for that amputee.

8. A ratchet or spiral ratchet screwdriver is easier than a rigid one though the method of using is the same; the split hook holds the shaft and the hand turns or pushes the screwdriver.

9. Large nails can be held in the Dorrance or Steeper adult split hook if it is turned points up, while small nails and panel pins can be held in tweezers held in the split hook. This demands considerable skill and is probably more often used as a training exercise rather than a practical method. Both the tweezers and the long-nosed pliers hold small nails and panel pins efficiently. An alternative method is to make a small hole first with a long nail or awl in which the small nail or panel pin can be placed, but this is essentially a one-handed method of achieving this skill and should be considered a last resort.

10. Finishing the article with paint or varnish should be done with the dominant hand regardless of whether this is the amputated limb or not. To expect an amputee to use his non-dominant prosthesis for a unilateral activity which is normally done with the dominant hand is not only unrealistic but can be harmful in that it attempts to establish false patterns of movement.

Metalwork

The degree to which this activity is used will depend on both the facilities available and the skill of the therapist. There is no reason why welding and metal lathe operation should not be included, but they will probably be beyond the scope of most departments. However, work with soft metals such as tin, copper and some alloys should be possible. Processes involved will be sawing, filing, use of tin snips and wire cutters, moulding by hammer and former, soldering and finishing, which can include enamelling as well as paint and varnish. All these activities demand the use of two hands and they can be easily graded by type of material, size of project and degree of complexity. An engineer's vice will be necessary and the material placed in it in the same way as for handling wood. For other processes proceed as follows:

1. When using a hacksaw it is normal to grasp the metal top with the non-dominant hand, so this is done with the split hook (rigid jaw on top).

2. Filing is also done with the sound hand, the split hook holding the file tip to give downward pressure.

3. Tin snips and wire cutters will be used in the sound hand with the material held in or steadied with the split hook.

4. Moulding in a former is usually of wire or metal strip. The unbent portion of the metal is held in the split hook while the intricate shaping is done with the sound hand. When moulding with a hammer the material being shaped will be held in the split hook. If the metal has been heated a split hook without rubber or plastic covers on the gripping surface should be used.

5. Finishing with paint or varnish should be done with the dominant hand.

6. Enamelling is usually an activity on its own and although the metal bases can be made from scratch they are more usually bought ready cut and finished. The process of enamelling can be made bimanual by sprinkling the enamel on to the metal with the sound hand and spreading with a wire held in the split hook. Articles should be placed on a tray for placing in the oven.

Light assembly work

This can include any constructional work involving the use of both hands. Placing of the materials to be assembled can encourage use and control of the split hook. A good exercise in assembly work is to have an electric circuit board which includes switches, bell and light run from a battery. This can be disconnected or wrongly wired for the amputee to rewire. A circuit diagram can be available to use if required. This can also provide a useful assessment not only in using a prosthesis but also in ability to follow a diagram, concentration and reasoning.

Technical drawing

This can easily be graded from the use of a short non-slip ruler (a strip of zinc plaster on the under surface of the ruler gives sufficient friction to prevent unintentional slip but still allows the ruler to be moved easily once the pressure is removed), to a plastic foot-rule used in conjunction with a set-square or protractor. It is bimanual and yet does not demand active prehension: a useful activity to intersperse with the more taxing exercises in cable control. The split hook should be positioned with hook points turned slightly inwards and the rigid jaw underneath so that pressure on the ruler can be easily maintained. Above-elbow amputees should have the elbow locked at 90° or less. If a metal hook is being used with no plastic or rubber cover to the outer surface a rubber thimble slipped over the lower hook point may be helpful in preventing slip between hook and ruler.

Typing

As has already been mentioned this is an excellent activity to teach control of the prosthesis in space. No special appliance is necessary when using the Dorrance or Steeper adult hooks as they point down-wards. A rubber thimble may be helpful to prevent the points slipping off the keys. Some amputees, particularly those with an above-elbow amputation, find it easier to use a rubber-tipped dowel or pencil in their split hook. This can be placed either vertically between the two gripping surfaces or sloping with the non-functional end resting on the cable level, as for writing (Fig. 29). Generally speaking it is not a good idea to give the amputee a typing appliance at this stage of his training as it requires him to adjust to a different total length of the prosthesis. Later, once the initial adjustment has been made, a typing peg can be useful to someone engaged in a lot of typing as it is simple and lightweight. The extent that typing can be used as a graded activity will depend on the level of amputation. A below-elbow

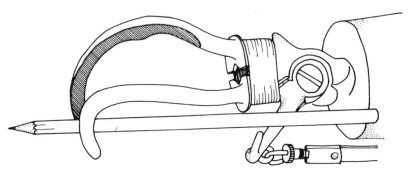

Fig. 29. Holding a pencil in a canted split hook with a three-point grasp.

amputee can progress quickly from space bar only to half the keys with his split hook, whilst an above-elbow will progress more slowly; a person with a through-shoulder amputation may never progress beyond using space bar or shift key.

Clerical activities

These should include writing for the amputee who has lost his dominant hand. A soft BB pencil or a fibre-tipped pen should be used and placed in the hook with the non-sharpened end resting on the cable lever (Fig. 29). The hook should be rotated so that the points are slightly medial and the tip of the pencil clearly visible to the writer. The amputee should be encouraged to practise large writing patterns, on unlined paper at first, as shown in the Marion Richardson writing books. Cursive writing is easier than printing individual letters because it does not demand continuous lifting of the pen or pencil tip from the paper. Writing with a prosthesis is more tiring than with a sound hand as it is not possible to rest the forearm on the table. Even if the amputee has practised writing pre-prosthetically he will have the extra weight of the prosthesis to control. Care must be taken to ensure that the writing surface is at the optimum height; ideally the relationship between writer and writing surface should be such that the elbow is slightly above the table when the shoulder is relaxed and the upper arm is held close to the body. Some amputees find it easier to write on a slightly tilted surface.

Other clerical activities could include sharpening pencils (hold the sharpener in the hook), folding a letter and inserting it into an envelope, wrapping and tying up a parcel, opening a letter using a knife held in split hook or hand, assembling looseleaf files, filing into a cabinet, using Sellotape, stapler, etc. For all these activities the prosthesis is used in a stabilizing and assistive role. These activities are all part of daily life and should not be restricted to those engaged in clerical-type work. Like technical drawing they can be usefully interspersed between more tiring cable-control activities, and, because they can be graded down to quite simple processes, they can be used early in training before a great deal of control has been learnt.

Gardening

This is easily graded from light to heavy work and so provides a good preparation and assessment for return to heavy work. It can range from indoor light gardening using a trowel, handfork or dibber for planting seedlings, cuttings, bulbs and pot plants through hoeing, raking and weeding outside to hedge trimming, lawn mowing and various grades of digging and shovelling. In the early stages of gardening the split hook will be found adequate but later, particularly for digging and shovelling, a speciality tool may be more suitable (see Figs 20 and 21).

When handling plants it is usually better to hold the plant in the sound hand and use the tool in the prosthesis. However, if gardening is started early in training the amputee may not have progressed sufficiently to be able to operate a split hook with a good grip. If this is so it may be necessary to adapt the handles of the tools to give a more positive grasp. This can be done either by padding the handle with felt or Rubazote to give a soft shaped gripping surface, or by filing a groove in the handle to allow the split hook to grip without slipping. The angle at which the tool is held will depend on whether the amputee is sitting or standing and should be adjusted so that the arm is used in a natural position to prevent back and shoulder strain. More suggestions for the method of using gardening tools and special appliances are included in the section on gardening as a hobby.

Sewing

For some women sewing is not only an essential activity but also an enjoyable one. However, it is not a particularly good activity for teaching active use of the split hook or prosthesis. A few processes require a fair degree of hand/hook/eye coordination but its chief value is in helping to establish a bimanual pattern of using the prosthesis and in proving to a person who needs to or wishes to sew that it is not beyond her capabilities. Embroidery using a ring can demand more active use of the split hook. Machine sewing improves general body coordination. For the below-elbow amputee a hand machine will demand the use of the prosthesis either for controlling the material or for turning the handle, while for the right above-elbow an electric or treadle machine is essential.

Plain sewing is best done at a table so that material can be arranged prior to placing it in the artificial hand or split hook. If the amputee is using a hand with a fabric or leather glove this should be removed, otherwise it may become sewn into the garment; when the hand has a cosmetic glove great care should be taken not to damage this with the needle. Generally speaking sewing, like most other activities, should be started with a split hook. A darning mushroom held in the split hook is good for holding the material when awkward sewing jobs are being tackled.

Knitting

This is a hobby of many women and some men which can be used to teach bimanual coordination of prosthesis and hand. Unless the amputee is already able to knit in the Continental fashion, the needle holding the stitches to be knitted is best held by the prosthesis so that the wool can be held in the sound hand. The right arm amputee should be taught to knit left-handed, a simple reversal of processes that only causes difficulty if a right-handed person casts on and starts the knitting, when the stitches must be reversed on the needle before the amputee begins to knit.

When using a split hook this should be turned so that the points face to the midline. It is simpler to hold the needles just between the gripping surfaces of the hook, otherwise the operating cord can become entangled in the knitting. Slight slip may be prevented by placing a large rubber band around the needle and the forearm section of the prosthesis. A knitting needle can usually be held in the standard hand fairly satisfactorily. It should be placed between the thumb and the first finger, with the knob end secured to the forearm with an elastic band.

Cooking and washing up

Simple domestic activities should be a routine part of all amputee training. They are excellent bimanual activities, can be graded in the degree of skill and coordination required, and washing and drying up the tea cups requires active use of the prosthesis in conjunction with the sound hand. When washing dishes it is best to use a mop or brush on a stick which can be held in the split hook (as for a pencil, Fig. 29); this minimizes the risk of water entering the wrist mechanism. For scouring saucepans the method is reversed, with the split hook being used to hold the saucepan handle (Fig. 30) or side while the scourer is used in the other hand. When drying a dish or cutlery, it is usually easier for the article to be placed in the split hook and dried with the sound hand but for flat dishes and cutlery the reverse is equally efficient.

Trays should have a raised handle large enough to accommodate the rigid finger of the split hook, which should be in the horizontal position. Saucers and plates should be held with the split hook at a similar angle so that the weight of the article being carried is supported on the rigid finger. When cooking it is important that the table is low enough for the amputee to work with the elbows extended to approximately 120°. This makes it easier for the amputee to handle the

objects being used and prevents fatigue. Generally speaking the prosthesis takes a non–dominant role, such as holding the bowl when
mixing (a damp cloth or non–slip mat under the bowl will help
stabilize it), the sieve when sifting and the saucepan when stirring.
When using a hand rotary whisk most arm amputees find it easiest to
hold the stabilizing handle with the prosthesis, though a few below-
elbow amputees who have lost their dominant hand prefer to do the
reverse. A rolling pin in which the centre portion spins on a dowel
connecting the handles allows for a firm grip with the split hook. Most
amputees find it quite practical to hold vegetables for paring in their
split hook, on a fork held in their split hook or on a spike board. A few
find it easier to use a potato peeler held in their split hook. A sharp-
pronged fork held in the split hook will make it easier to hold meat and
vegetables steady while chopping with the other hand. Sharp kitchen
knives should not be held in the prosthesis. Not only might the
amputee's only sound hand be unintentionally damaged (as when
using woodwork tools) but also, if the amputee is distracted by such
things as a child crying or a telephone ringing, she might forget that

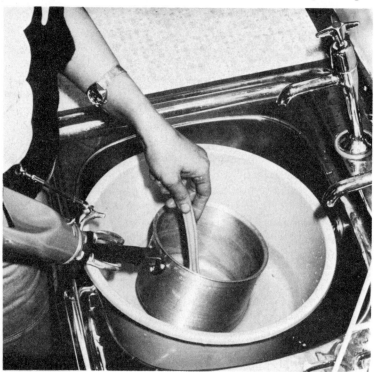

Fig. 30. An above–elbow amputee cleaning a saucepan.

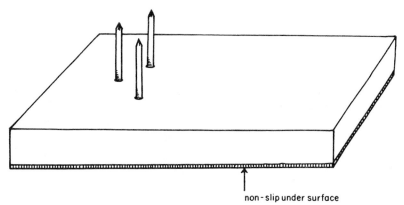

non - slip under surface

Fig. 31. A spiked board for stabilizing bread, meat or vegetables ready for cutting.

she is holding the knife and so create a hazard for others in the vicinity. A spike board (Fig. 31) is an invaluable kitchen aid for chopping vegetables and meat and for cutting bread. It is easily made from a piece of 1 cm (0.5 in) board and aluminium nails, and should have a non-slip undersurface. Handling casseroles, pie dishes and cake tins can be difficult with a split hook so these should be put on a flat baking tray before placing in the oven. Fortunately most modern ovens have shelves which can be partly drawn out to allow the cook to inspect, stir or turn round baking without having to lift it out.

Games and sports

Billiards, cricket and table tennis have been mentioned as possible games to use in teaching bimanual use of the prosthesis. There are, of course, many others. Cards and darts are two indoor games within the scope of most people. In all these games the prosthesis takes the non-dominant role. When playing billiards the split hook or palm of the prosthetic hand (palm facing up) makes a useful rest. When using a cricket bat the split hook can be used on the top or shaft of the bat, though serious players will find the spade grip (see Fig. 20) more satisfactory. In table tennis the ball can be held and thrown with split hook or hand (palm side up). A hand of cards can be quite satisfactorily held in either split hook or prosthetic hand, though care needs to be taken not to let one's opponent see the cards! Playing cards is a useful way to teach fine control of the operating cord, as only slight tension has to be placed on it to allow one card to be withdrawn without the others falling to the floor. This also applies to darts held in the split hook, though if the standard prosthetic hand is worn the darts will rest between the thumb and the first finger without activating the thumb.

81

Games have the additional psychological advantage that they encourage amputees to compete and learn from each other in a relaxed setting. The skills learnt will make it easier for them to become integrated into their home community.

Although an attempt has been made in this section to give the amputee and the therapist ideas both on how to tackle a task and how to make it a useful therapeutic medium, there are many ways of doing things. There is no 'right' way of achieving a goal, only safe ways and means of using activities for a specific purpose; in this case to learn to use the prosthesis in a relaxed and natural fashion. This will often influence the choice of method or medium selected at a particular stage of training, although there is little point in expecting an amputee to tackle a task in an uncomfortable or awkward fashion purely to give him practice in using his prosthesis. Far better to choose another activity which demands the desired pattern of movements, is within the degree of skill already learnt and achieves a recognizable goal.

ACTIVITIES OF DAILY LIVING

In its broadest sense this covers everything that one does in the course of the day. However, for the purposes of this section it is used in its narrower meaning to cover those parts of activities essential to one's personal care, such as dressing, washing and eating, which are sometimes a problem for the single arm amputee.

Dressing

By the time the amputee is fitted with his prosthesis he has usually mastered the art of putting on and taking off his clothes without his prosthesis but often still has difficulties with fastenings, the main problem being to hold two pieces of material under tension to button, hook or press-stud them together. Pulling up zips when the bottom needs holding, as in an anorak, and tying shoelaces and ties can sometimes prove difficult also.

At first dressing and undressing seem more difficult when wearing the prosthesis than it was without and a little help and instruction may prevent an initial discarding of the prosthesis as being more of a hindrance than a help. The amputee should be encouraged to put on all lower garments before putting on the prosthesis, i.e. pants, tights, socks, trousers or skirt. When putting on shirts or dresses the prosthesis should be put into the sleeve first, then the garment taken over the head and lastly the other arm inserted. This method is usually satisfactory for a below-elbow amputee wearing his prosthesis. Some above-elbow and most through-shoulder amputees find it easier to put the shirt on to the prosthesis before putting on the prosthesis. Ladies should avoid dresses with limited openings and many find either a front opening or a zip down the back the easiest as they allow plenty of room to manoeuvre, although zips at the back can be difficult to fasten even with a zip aid.

The fastenings that most commonly cause difficulty are those at the waist, where tension has to be maintained on both sides of the fastening. An inconspicuous loop of tape or self material (taken from the hem or inside a pocket) stitched to the side opposite to the prosthesis will enable the amputee to insert the tips of the hook to pull without relying on the tension of the grasp (Fig. 32). A similar loop can be stitched at the bottom of zips if fastening these is a problem. Hooks are usually easier than press-studs to fasten at the waist. If conventional waist fastenings cannot be managed, Velcro (see Fig. 6) can be used, but as this necessitates adapting every pair of trousers or skirt it should be a last resort.

Ties are easily managed with practice though a few men prefer to use the clip-on varieties. The underneath end should be held in the split hook (above-elbow amputees should lock the elbow in full flexion) while the knot is tied with the sound hand. If the tie slips out of the hook a small loop can be stitched under the narrow end for the hook to slip into. Many ties have a label conveniently placed for this purpose!

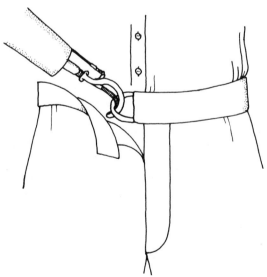

Fig. 32. A loop on the waistband allows the hook to exert maximum tension when fastening.

A few through-shoulder and forequarter amputees cannot master this technique and if this is a problem they may prefer to use a one-handed technique, securing the narrow end of the tie in a chest drawer or with a loop on to a trouser button.

Fastening the *cuff button* of the sound arm presents a problem for the arm amputee unable to slip his hand through the fastened cuff. There are three possible ways of overcoming this:

1. Sew the cuff button on with elastic thread so that it is possible to push the hand through the fastened cuff.

2. Use expanding cuff links for the same effect.

3. Use a button hook (see Fig. 76). These are available as standard issue from the limb-fitting centre stores in the United Kingdom. The shaft of the button hook is held in the split hook; the wire inserted through the buttonhole and looped on to the button so that the hook pulls the button through the buttonhole when it is withdrawn. Once the button is fastened, the button hook is pushed forward so that the button slips out through the wider part of the wire loop.

Shoelaces seem to some amputees to be an insurmountable problem and though it needs practice to learn to fasten securely with either one hand or hand and prosthesis, this is not all that difficult. A below-elbow amputee should have no problem in learning to tie a shoelace with hook and hand. Some above-elbow amputees and most through-shoulder and forequarter amputees find it much easier to learn to fasten them with one hand. It is best to practise first with a shoe on the table, having made sure that the laces are of good length. A practice shoe with two different coloured laces knotted together before insertion into the shoe ensures a good length for practising, and has the advantage that it is easy to differentiate between the laces. Once the bow can be tied on the practice shoe, then the amputee can practise on his own shoe (off his foot) progressing finally to tying it on his foot. A number of fastening methods are available:

1. Using hook and hand. Once the knot has been tied, a loop is made and held at the base in the split hook; the second lace is then passed round this loop and tucked under to form the second loop. The amputee then leaves go of the first loop (held in his split hook) and grasps the end of the second loop with his split hook; at the same time he takes hold of the tip of the first loop with his sound hand. He is then in a position to pull the loops tight. It is often necessary in the early stages of practising to stop before finally tightening to make the loops smaller to prevent the ends pulling through and making a knot.

2. Using one hand only. The method of tying the bow as described above but, instead of holding the loop in the split hook it is held against

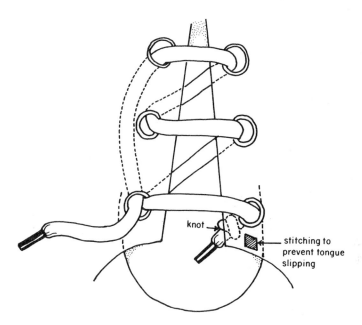

knot

stitching to
prevent tongue
slipping

Fig. 33. A one-handed method of lacing a shoe.

the shoe upper with the second finger, while the second lace is
positioned over it with the index finger and thumb; the loop is then
held between the third finger and thumb while the lace is tucked
behind and through to form the second loop with the index finger.
Once the two loops are formed it is a simple matter to hold one
between the thumb and third finger and the other between the index
and second finger to tighten. Practice is needed to be able to secure a
shoe tightly with this method, particularly if using the non–dominant
hand. Flat shoelaces are much easier than round ones.

3. Should the amputee find both these methods unsatisfactory he
can try lacing the shoe from the top to the toe (Fig. 33). There must be a
knot in the starting end of the lace and he finishes by threading the lace
under the lacing on one side and up through the top hole. With this
method of lacing he can loosen the laces sufficiently to slip his foot into
the shoe and then tighten working from the top to the toe, finally
taking up the slack with the loose end. This can then either be knotted
in a half–bow around the top lace or tucked into the side of the shoe.
The tongue should be stitched to the upper at one side to prevent it
slipping when the foot is inserted.

4. Another alternative to tying bows is to use either elastic shoelaces
or round elastic as laces. This converts laced shoes into slip-ons.

Careful choice of clothing can often do away with the necessity to adapt. Points to look for are:

1. Trousers and skirts with flat trouser hooks and bar.
2. Fastenings at the front or on the non-amputated side.
3. Shirts, blouses and dresses with extra roominess at the back to allow for scapula movement when activating the operating cord.
4. Raglan or dolman sleeves rather than tight set-in sleeves.
5. Buttonholes on knitted garments big enough for the button to slip through easily with one hand.
6. Shoes that slip on or fasten with buckles or zips. If using laces choose flat laces rather than round ones.
7. Corsets with zips, or even better a pull-tight hook fastening like that fitted on some surgical corsets. Tight roll-ons are very difficult to pull on with one hand. Back suspenders are difficult and if the amputee must wear a belt they should position the back suspenders as near the outside as possible. Tights are much easier to manage and worn in conjunction with a pantie-girdle are often quite satisfactory even for the woman with the 'fuller figure'.
8. Brassières with elastic shoulder straps are not only more comfortable under a prosthesis but also easier to put on. Fasten the bra in front, turn it around so that the fastening is at the back, then slip first the sound arm and then the stump into the shoulder straps.

Washing, hair care and cutting nails

Most washing can be done with one hand after a little practice. Some arm amputees have difficulty at first putting soap on a flannel or sponge, washing and drying their sound arm and washing their backs. Most people who are restricted to washing with one hand find that they can put soap on a flannel by placing it across their knee, below-elbow stump or the side of the basin before rubbing soap on to it; others find a sponge easier to stabilize. An alternative is to have a towelling mitt on the sound hand, which can be rubbed on to soap held firmly on a soap holder (a little octopus soap holder which has suckers on both sides is available at most chemists). To wash the sound hand lay the flannel across the below-elbow stump, side of the basin or knee if in the bath and rub arm on to it. A nailbrush can either be held in the split hook, or attached to the side of the basin or bath with suction pads. Washing the back is most easily done with a long-handled bath brush or loofah. If drying the sound arm is a problem the amputee should try hanging a towel from an elastic loop on to a hook at shoulder level or higher when he should be able to dry his arm by rubbing it against the towel while holding it in the hand.

Many women find washing and setting their hair with one hand extremely difficult. Some people do have much more difficult hair to manage than others, so some women may prefer to have their hair done regularly at the hairdresser. However, if it is possible to keep hair reasonably short there is no reason why the single arm amputee cannot manage it herself. Washing hair is easiest done over the bath with a spray attachment on the taps. Partially dry the hair before attempting to set it. Spiked rollers are the easiest to put in with one hand and can be held in place with the stump or split hook while inserting pin or clip to secure. It is probably easier to practise this on someone else before attempting to set one's own hair.

It is obviously going to be impossible to cut the nails of the sound hand with scissors, so nail clippers, a nail file or emery board must be used. A nail file or emery board can be held in either the split hook or prosthetic hand, and is probably the easiest method if done regularly. Nail clippers should be secured to a board so that the base is held firmly and the clippers protrude over the edge; the nails can then be cut by placing the board with clippers attached on a table and pressing down on the clippers with split hook, prosthetic hand or stump.

Use of cutlery

Arm amputees with a North American upbringing score here for they need only learn to cut their meat and from then on can eat one-handed without feeling different. However, in Europe the custom is to use cutlery in both hands throughout the meal. Whether the amputee decides to be European or North American is a matter of personal choice.

When using a knife and fork throughout the meal it is easier to hold the knife in the prosthesis so that the fork, which has to be lifted and

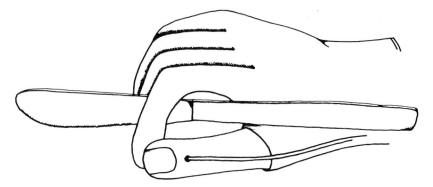

Fig. 34. The position of the knife in a prosthetic hand to give a firm grasp for cutting.

rotated to reach the mouth, can be held in the sound hand. The knife can be used quite efficiently in a prosthetic hand with rigid fingers (Fig. 34) or is equally satisfactory when placed in a split hook as for a pencil (see Fig. 29). The split hook or hand should be rotated so that the knife blade has the cutting edge at right angles to the plate. As for all activities carried out seated at a table it is important that the amputee is sitting high enough for the elbow to be clear of the table top when he first attempts this activity. Otherwise he will find either that the knife is cutting the side of the plate, rather than its contents, or that he has to abduct his arm to such an extent that he knocks his neighbour off his seat. Practice with a stale piece of bread or plasticine is a good idea before attempting this at a mealtime. Yeast buns or rolls are of a good consistency for cutting without disintegrating and can also be eaten with enjoyment. If the arm amputee decides to eat 'American style' he can hold either the knife or the fork in his prosthesis, for he will then lay down the knife once the food is cut up and eat with a fork only held in his sound hand. A fork is placed in the split hook or hand in a similar way to the knife, but because it is broad side down the hand or split hook will be rotated so that the prosthetic thumb or cable lever is on top. Some amputees find it more satisfactory to place the fork between the third and fourth finger rather than the first and second when using a fork in the prosthetic hand. If using a spoon and fork for eating the fork will be placed as just described for its purpose is that of a pusher rather than for taking the food to the mouth.

RELEVANCE TO WORK AND HOBBIES

Most single arm amputees are young males of working age who lose their hands in an accident. They are keen to return to work and continue with their chosen hobbies. Occasionally this is not possible, or only partly so, because employers and insurers have regulations which prevent a handicapped person doing certain jobs. More often neither the amputee or the employer think that a particular job is possible for an arm amputee. Very few jobs are beyond the capabilities of a single arm amputee, particularly if his amputation is below the elbow and of his non-dominant hand. The higher the level of amputation the greater the challenge.

The amputee who wants to return to his former job should explore every avenue to see if it is possible. There have been pilots who have returned to flying, doctors who have continued in medicine and printers who have returned to their trade. Many more have had promotion to positions supervising the skills they previously performed. Others have chosen re-training and have become welders, paint sprayers or draughtsmen. No arm amputee should assume that his working days are over when he loses a hand.

During the early stages of training it is necessary to use certain types of activities to give the arm amputee practice in operating and controlling his prostheses. But in the later stages it is often possible to simulate work and hobby situations so that training begins to have a realistic setting. An arm amputee who uses specialist tools should be asked to bring these to his training session. He can then try them out in the relaxed atmosphere of the department without the interested, but critical, eyes of employers and workmates. Using a different method or another appliance will often overcome any difficulty and when confident in his own ability the amputee can demonstrate his capabilities at work. Sometimes it is not possible to bring the tools to the department or may be the worker is handling large machinery. This is where general practice in handling woodwork and metalwork tools is an advantage and if the department has access to heavier machinery, such as lathes and power drills, the amputee will gain in confidence. Occasionally it is possible to arrange with the employers for the arm amputee to try out machinery when the factory is closed. A work visit can then be arranged with either occupational therapist, technician or technical officer.

Time should be spent discussing hobbies as well as jobs. With increasing leisure and early retirement the ability to continue with satisfying hobbies helps to keep a person mentally healthy. Driving, home repairs and decorating, gardening, car maintenance, knitting, dressmaking and music are among the more common hobbies.

Participation in sports is often important too and there is usually no reason why a single arm amputee should not continue with a sport which he enjoys. Obviously he will be handicapped in some, but while he may be unable to compete in competitions he is unlikely to be prevented from enjoying the sport. In many sports arm amputees can compete on nearly equal terms, their amputations being little handicap once they have developed skill with the appropriate appliance. The more common sports enjoyed by arm amputees are fishing, football, swimming, skin-diving, cricket, tennis, badminton, golf, shooting, sailing, ski-ing, riding and fencing. But many others are possible, so no arm amputee should assume that he cannot continue with a favourite sport because he has lost an arm.

Driving

Most people want to be able to drive even if they are at that time unable to own a car. For the single below-elbow amputee this should cause few problems. With the recommended driving cup appliance (p. 56) and a ball clamped to the steering wheel he will be able to both steer and change gear with his prosthesis. He should avoid a car with steering column gear change or handbrake on his amputated side. If buying a car it is worth considering where the indicators, light switches and windscreen wiper switches are positioned, for it is both easier and safer if these are on the non-amputated side of the steering column. The person with an above-elbow prosthesis may find changing gear with his prosthesis difficult and so should choose a car with a gear lever on the non-amputated side or a car with automatic gear change. The handbrake should be on the non-amputated side but this can be moved quite easily, unlike the gear box. Through-shoulder and forequarter amputees should not attempt to use the prosthesis for more than steadying the wheel and so to all intents and purposes they should modify their car to be driven with one hand. This means that an automatic gear change is advisable and the handbrake and all controls should be on the non-amputated side. The British School of Motoring have in their main office in Knightsbridge an experienced team to advise on modification to different makes of cars. However, a visit should only be necessary for a single arm amputee if he is unable to get the help he needs from the technical officer at his local limb-fitting centre.

Home repairs and maintenance

The amputee will already have practised handling carpentry and metalwork tools during training in control of the prosthesis. Painting is basically a one-handed job but paper-hanging is more difficult. However, it should be within the competence of a below-elbow amputee. He should use his split hook and start with short lengths of paper of medium thickness. When plastering, or using cement, he will hold the float or hawk which holds the plaster or cement in his split hook and spread with the float or trowel in his sound hand.

Gardening

The keen gardener should try out the spade grip and William C hook (see Figs 20 and 21) as well as his split hook for the basic gardening activities, i.e. a spade or fork, a long-handled tool such as hoe or rake, shears, lawn mower and small fork or trowel. Some people find the small tools easier to manage if the handle is inserted into a hammer holder. The spade grip can be used either on the top of the tool (Fig. 20) or on the shaft, the latter being more common for long-handled tools.

When hoeing and raking the amputee should be encouraged to try with the split hook both below and above the sound hand, as it may be easier for him to control the tool in a different way from that used before he lost his hand. For some the pattern of movement is very firmly established and these people find it easier to continue with the same method though maybe less efficiently than before. Garden shears can be used with a strong gripping split hook or a spade grip; the above-elbow amputee will have to lock his elbow and lateral to give sufficient force and control for this activity. A split hook is usually satisfactory for a wheelbarrow, though some amputees find a bolt dropped through a hole at the end of the handle, so that it provides a stop, helpful when moving a laden barrow. The handles of lawn mowers vary considerably in shape and height so it is difficult to be specific about how they should be controlled. A split hook is usually satisfactory on a hand mower, with maybe extra padding on the handle to prevent slip.

Some amputees find it easier to clamp an appliance such as a universal toolholder, A and W toolholder or hammer holder on to the handle of a push-type lawn mower while others manage quite efficiently with a split hook. It depends very much on the individual amputee and type of lawn mower. Judiciously placed padding on the handle will often be sufficient to give a better grip and prevent sideways slip of the split hook. Motor mowers should have their clutch and throttle controls positioned so that they can be operated by the sound hand and the clamping-on of an appliance should be avoided so that the handle may be released quickly in an emergency. Many people find a driving cup and ball satisfactory while others are happy working with their split hook. For indoor gardening a dibber or short length of dowel is often a useful tool which can be easily held in the split hook.

Car maintenance

Part of an old car engine is sometimes available in an occupational therapy department for practice in handling spanners and wrenches. If not, a bicycle or lawn mower can usually be acquired for this purpose.

Spanners must be put into the split hook so that force can be exerted. One end must rest against the operating cord lever or the body of the hook. The first method is similar to the placing of a knife or pencil (see Fig. 29) but with the split hook turned so that the points face medially. The second method uses the curve of the hook to give stability. Pliers (p. 58) can sometimes prove more effective for this type of activity. If possible appliances should be lent to the amputee to try out at home before a final choice is made.

Knitting

This has already been covered in bimanual activities. However one-handed knitting, using a clamp on a table to hold the left hand needle or tucking this needle under the arm, is possible.

Dressmaking

This assumes the ownership of a sewing machine and an electric or treadle machine will certainly take much of the labour out of dressmaking for the arm amputee. It is easier to pin out the pattern and cut on a smooth hard surface, which will not be easily damaged by pins; scrubbed deal is ideal but formica is satisfactory although a little slippery. Left-handed scissors are now available or battery-operated ones may be easier for a person who has lost a dominant hand. Tacking is tedious and, except for setting in sleeves and gathers, pins are often adequate. A machine which will hem, neaten edges and buttonhole is a great help to an arm amputee and would be a good investment for a keen dressmaker.

Music

For many people music means listening to music on record or tape and going to concerts, but some like to make music in however simple a way. The piano is probably the most commonly played instrument and unfortunately it is perhaps the least suitable for the arm amputee. The musician will be limited to single notes or two note chords with his amputated arm. Some people find a typing peg or two-pronged office appliance easier to use than the split hook or hand. String instruments are easier to play. With the addition of a moulded block to fit into the palm, the bow can be held in the prosthetic hand. A pick for playing the guitar and other plucked string instruments can be held in either the split hook or hand, though some below-elbow amputees prefer to strap it directly to their stump. If the left hand has been lost the instrument will have to be re-strung for left-hand playing. Many brass instruments are very suitable for they can be held with the prosthesis or rested on the back of a chair and need only one hand for fingering. A harmonica can be held in a split hook or artificial hand (Fig. 35), between shortened arms or mounted on a stand. Percussion instruments are possible, but to get a good sound the hammer or stick must be held very loosely in the prosthesis. A spring or length of flexible material inserted into the shaft of the hammer makes it easier to achieve the correct tone when playing the xylophone.

Sports

Of the sports mentioned, football needs no additional appliance and is possibly better played either without the prosthesis or with just the prosthesis and no terminal device. This will depend on whether the stump needs the protection of the prosthesis or whether it is a hindrance to free movement and a danger to other players. The same can apply to some other sports and will largely depend on the level of amputation and the extent to which the amputee finds the prosthesis a help with the sport.

Swimming should always be without the prosthesis unless a special suction watertight prosthesis has been made specifically for this purpose. These are not normally available or necessary for swimming to be enjoyed. Most swimmers find it easier to do a sidestroke, modified

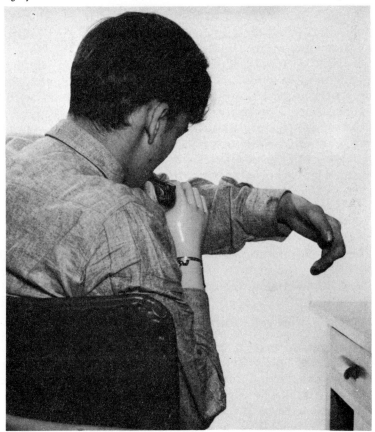

Fig. 35. A harmonica may be held in the prosthetic hand if it is not possible to bring the other hand to the mouth.

crawl or backstroke. A few below-elbow amputees find that a foot flipper, strapped to the stump, with the elbow in the heel position, helps them swim in a straight line and underwater. Skin divers can have their wet-suit adapted by the manufacturers to fit over the stump.

A spade grip is helpful for holding and controlling a cricket bat and is usually placed on the top of the bat (see Fig. 20) with the sound hand on the shaft. A few right arm amputees find it difficult to reverse their batting action and prefer to have the spade grip on the shaft or to use a split hook.

Tennis and badminton need no special appliance and are often easier to play one-handed. The ball is held between the fourth finger and the thenar eminence while the racquet is held between the first two fingers and thumb. A little practice is needed to coordinate the serve but this is soon mastered.

Some golf players choose to play one-handed but a below-elbow amputee should find the golf appliance both satisfactory and a help with maintaining balance and swing.

There are also special appliances for fishing, sailing, ski-ing and riding but for these sports many amputees use their split hook, hand or stump. It very much depends on the level at which one is participating. Small boat sailing is probably better done without the prosthesis for if the boat capsizes the prosthesis could be a hindrance to swimming. Ski-ing without a prosthesis means using only one stick, which can upset balance, but experts often ski with no sticks. Riding can be done one-handed, but again balance is upset, particularly if jumping is to be included. Fencing is a one-handed sport and, once balance has been mastered, can be, and has been, taken to Olympic standards.

Solving the problem of returning to work and continuing with hobbies is often the most stimulating part of the therapist's job. It is an exercise in communication, imagination, adaptability and originality. The solutions are sometimes unorthodox, like making a glove with a pocket to hold fledgling pigeons while they are ringed.

Further rehabilitation and return to work

Some arm amputees are either unable to return to their previous job or do not wish to do so. Even if they have definite plans for future employment or training, they are advised in the United Kingdom to register at their local Job Centre or Employment Service Agency as a disabled person. They then have the service of the Disablement Resettlement Officer (DRO) to help them find a new job, to arrange a course of rehabilitation at an Employment Rehabilitation Centre (ERC) or training at a Skills Centre.

A disabled person, without a skill, is at a disadvantage in open employment, so the arm amputee without either job or qualifications would be wise to take advantage of the opportunity to train at a Skills Centre. There is quite a range of courses from clerical to welding and tailoring to horticulture. Some centres have only selected courses so it may be necessary for the candidate to travel to another part of the country to pursue his chosen career. Popular courses for single arm amputees are welding and paint spraying, though they are by no means limited to these. If a person has been unemployed for some time and is out of the habit of regular work, rehabilitation at an ERC will help him re-establish work patterns and build up both his physical and

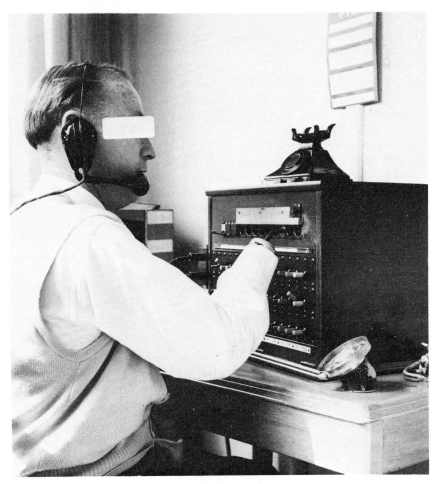

Fig. 36. A blind double below-elbow amputee employed as a switchboard operator.

mental stamina. Sometimes this is all that is necessary to bridge the gap between hospital and work. Many people go straight from the ERC into open employment without further training.

Re-training for arm amputees is not limited to government re-settlement schemes. Many amputees go into open training schemes and apprenticeships. Each individual will need a different rehabilitation and training programme. Many hospitals and rehabilitation centres in the United Kingdom have regular visits from their local DRO. Continuity from hospital to employment is maintained and the patient knows what is to be the next stage of his rehabilitation before he leaves hospital. If no such system is established it is the responsibility of the occupational therapist to see that this referral is made and that the arm amputee is aware of the various possibilities open to him. He should never be discharged from training into a vacuum. At least an outline programme must be established. There is a standard form for referral of amputees to the Department of Employment. It must be signed by the amputee and then given to the limb-fitting surgeon for completion. If an amputee has had no such referral he can get the form from his local employment office or job centre. It is helpful to the limb-fitting surgeon completing the form if he has a report from the therapist responsible for training. This should cover the areas which are of interest to the Department of Employment to ensure that the potential of the amputee using the prosthesis is fully exploited for work.

Occupational therapy departments should have a wide range of activities to be used therapeutically. It may, however, be necessary to adapt the department so that it can be used as a dissecting room for a budding biologist, a kitchen for a young baker to practise using a forcing bag or a quiet corner for the priest to practise handling chalice and salver. The purpose is to give people the opportunity to learn how to make the most of their prostheses and to understand its full possibilities and its shortcomings. In fact, to learn how to live with their prostheses.

References

Fishman, S. (1959) Amputee needs, frustrations and behaviour. *Rehab. Lit.*, 20, 322–9.

Richardson, M. (1935) *Writing Patterns*. London: University of London Press.

CHAPTER 13

Learning to Live with Two Artificial Arms

Psychological effect of losing two hands

To lose one hand is a profound shock, to lose both hands is a disaster; it must seem like the end of a meaningful life. Initially the double arm amputee is completely dependent for all his most intimate personal needs and at this stage can see no possible way to personal or financial independence. His self-esteem is shattered and he feels like a helpless cripple. No longer will he be able to fondle his loved ones, feel or gesticulate. As well as the body being maimed and manipulative skills lost, the means of emotional expression and communication are gone.

The accident of losing both hands affects not only the amputee but also his whole family, who thus become important elements in his successful rehabilitation. Their problems of adjustment must also be considered if they are to become helpful members of the rehabilitation team. Without their positive help rehabilitation will be a slower and a longer process; it may even fail to reach a successful conclusion. To walk the tight-rope of loving, caring and helping and still be able to withdraw physical help and support when necessary is a very difficult task. Yet without this understanding and skill in those closest to the double arm amputee, all the expertise and training of the professionals can fail to give him true independence.

The respect and status accorded to a person by his family, his friends and the community in which he lives often reflect his quality of life and this can be threatened by amputation. The double arm amputee's appraisal of this respect will be dependent on his own feelings about handicapped persons prior to his amputation. His perception of his amputation and its affect on his ability to satisfy his needs will ultimately determine his ability to adjust to living with two artificial arms. The single arm amputee frequently experiences frustration but the person who has lost both hands is frustrated constantly. Physical function is perhaps the easiest need to tackle but also one where compromises have to be made. The need to look normal, to be complete, can unfortunately never be fully satisfied. To wear two artificial arms constantly requires acceptance of a degree of discomfort and time for adjustment. The physical effort involved in doing the simplest activity is many times greater with prostheses than with one's own hands. Lower standards of achievement may have to be accepted initially and limitations placed on the areas where an acceptable standard of achievement is worth the effort involved. The desire to be economically secure and able to earn one's own living with two arm prostheses limits the opportunities available and can force the double arm amputee to do a job for which he has no inclination but which offers financial security.

The first compromise the double arm amputee will be asked to make is the acceptance of split hooks rather than hands. They are easier to learn to control and use than are mechanical hands and so offer a better chance of achieving early independence. Preparation for this should be by discussion, explanation and reassurance that hands will be available if wanted later.

In the United Kingdom the double arm amputee will normally be trained with two Dorrance split hooks. All skills should be taught using these and only in exceptional circumstances should alternative appliances or mechanical hands be considered. A few double arm amputees opt for one hand at a later stage but rarely does a double arm amputee want to sacrifice the independence possible when wearing the split hook for two useless cosmetic hands or the increased weight and comparative clumsiness of mechanical hands. A few long-established users of mechanical hands may dispute this and should a double arm amputee wish to try a mechanical hand once he has completed his initial training with split hooks, it should be possible to arrange this. In the first half of the twentieth century it was the practice in the United Kingdom to give double arm amputees a case full of specially designed appliances, one for each activity he wished to do, but this is no longer encouraged as it never gave any degree of real independence. A double arm amputee can be completely independent with two Dorrance split hooks if he has sufficient practice and training in the use of these. The provision of a special appliance should be the exception rather than the rule.

Initial independence

The discovery that there are some things that one can do helps in the adjustment to amputation. Amongst the first things a double arm amputee should be taught is to feed himself and to write. Learning the skills of prehension and fine control can follow once the double arm amputee has realized that the prostheses have some potential for him.

SELF–FEEDING

If there has been a delay between amputation and referral for prostheses the amputee should have been taught to feed himself and to write using a gauntlet as described on p. 15. The skill will then only have to be transferred to the prosthesis. This entails deciding on the best angle for the spoon and fork and the best height for the table, as well as adjustment to the extra length and weight of the prosthesis.

If the double arm amputee has one stump longer than the other he should use this arm for self-feeding regardless of dominance, unless the difference in length is minimal or there is some other disabling factor to consider. Should he have a through-wrist or partially mutilated hand he will still have forearm movement, which will make loading the spoon and keeping it level much easier. If his amputation is below the elbow he still has his own elbow movement for bringing the spoon or fork to his mouth and unrestricted shoulder movement, so that he can compensate for the lost forearm movement by using shoulder rotation. The double above-elbow amputee may need a self-righting or floating spoon when he starts to eat runny foods though he should be able to manage an ordinary fork held in his split hook.

It is probably easiest to start self-feeding with a fork to avoid the additional problem of keeping the spoon level while learning the first skills of picking up food and taking it to the mouth. A food that is easily speared and does not crumble should be chosen. Sausages, roast potatoes, slices of apple and banana are all excellent. A small piece of metal tube soldered under the handle of the fork where it is to be gripped prevents the fork being knocked out of alignment or accidentally dropped during the early stages when there may be a force of

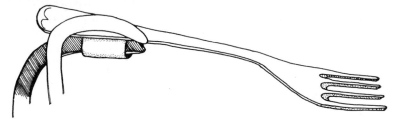

Fig. 37. A tube soldered on to a fork helps to give a firm grasp with the split hook.

only 1 kg (1–2 lb) in the grasp of the split hook. The lower finger of the hook is then inserted into this tube when holding the fork (Fig. 37). A similar tube can be soldered to a dessertspoon for training purposes. Once the amputee has mastered the skill of loading the spoon and fork and can open his split hook with three bands in position he should not need this aid. When using a fork for spearing food a flat plate is quite satisfactory but when using a spoon, a deep plate is better. Should the amputee have difficulty loading the spoon a special plate with one straight edge or a plateguard clipped to a flat plate should prove helpful (Fig. 38). A non–slip mat will prevent the plate slipping on a shiny

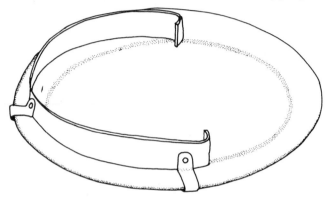

Fig. 38. A plate guard clipped to a flat plate.

surface. If none is available a damp cloth or even slightly wetting the tablecloth (providing the table is not polished) will help to stabilize the plate.

The double above–elbow amputee who needs to use a floating spoon can have this plugged directly into his prosthesis in place of the split hook. This makes self-feeding easier but should be considered only as a stage in learning. Continued with indefinitely it will prevent the amputee returning to full independence. A special spoon, which will probably need to be put in and taken out of the prosthesis by someone else, does not encourage independent feeding, but can give a degree of independence to the more severely handicapped who is unable to use ordinary cutlery. The floating spoon should be attached to a flat adaptor so that it can be rotated by pressure against the plate or in the mouth. The sprung-loaded balls in the wrist unit should provide sufficient friction to prevent unwanted movement.

At this stage drinking is best continued with a straw until the split hook has a sufficiently strong grip for the amputee to feel confident holding a cup (see Fig. 42).

To be able to sign one's own name and communicate by writing is a valued skill. Fortunately it is one of the easier skills for the double arm amputee to re-learn, although it can be tiring if too much is undertaken. The prolific writer will find a typewriter a great help.

The method of learning to write has already been described (pp. 14, 77). The double arm amputee may need the paper secured to a board in the early stages but otherwise he should proceed as for the single arm amputee who has lost his dominant hand. Short periods of writing interspersed with other different activities will prevent fatigue.

Learning control of the prostheses

The technique of learning control of a prosthesis has already been described for the single arm amputee (p. 66). The double arm amputee must learn more precise control before purposeful activities can be started because there is no sound hand to do three-quarters of the work. More time will have to be spent on specific activities to teach this control. Planning the training programme is of vital importance so that new skills, within the amputee's competence, can be introduced on days when progress seems to be at a standstill and the patient appears discouraged and depressed.

Realistic activities of importance to the amputee should be introduced as soon as possible. The smoker can learn to open a flip-top cigarette packet, partially pull out a cigarette, pick up the packet and take it to his mouth so that he is able to withdraw the cigarette with his lips. He can be encouraged to keep his money in a tray purse so that he can shake out the coins and pick up the appropriate one for purchases in the canteen. Practice in fastening buttons on a button board or on an old cardigan laid on a table may seem more purposeful to an adult than posting shapes through a posting box.

PUTTING ON AND TAKING OFF THE PROSTHESES

For the first few days the double arm amputee will be helped, but as he is dependent on his prostheses for the simplest of activities it is vital for him to be able to put on and take off his prostheses independently and with ease. To do this he should hang his prostheses by the shoulder straps, either from two hooks at shoulder level or on the back of a chair facing the seat so that he can sit on the chair when puting them on. He should insert the longer stump first, unless one is above-elbow and the other below-elbow when the above-elbow prosthesis is put on first. As the shoulder straps are held at shoulder level or above, he can shrug his shoulders in under these straps while removing them from the hooks or chairback. The straps joining a pair of above-elbow prostheses usually cause no difficulty, but many people find the appendages very confusing when one or two below-elbow prostheses are worn. If the appendages are getting twisted, it is worth marking the front two shoulder straps so that they are easily identified. The below-elbow stump must go under these and behind the V-straps joining them to the socket (see Fig. 23), while all the other straps should be behind the stump.

All prostheses should be worn over a cotton or woollen sock shaped to fit smoothly over the stump. These are available in the United Kingdom from the limb-fitting centres. A double below-elbow amputee should have no bother putting on his stump socks and keeping them in position while putting on his prostheses. For an above-elbow amputee this is more of a problem and many find it easier to wear a T-shirt with the sleeves stitched with a flat seam to form a smooth covering to the stump. If the sleeve is not long enough to do this a cotton stump sock can be stitched into the end of the sleeve to replace it. A T-shirt has the additional advantage of providing protection across the back and shoulders from the friction of the appendages. Most women prefer a cosy top because it is cut lower in the front than a T-shirt.

Once the prostheses are on, the double arm amputee with at least one below-elbow prosthesis should have no difficulty in putting on a shirt or loose-fitting sweater, but the double above-elbow amputee would be wise to put his shirt on to his prostheses before putting them on so that he only has the front fastening to contend with (p. 109).

EVALUATING THE DEGREE OF INDEPENDENCE POSSIBLE

Complete independence is always the ultimate goal in rehabilitation, but it is unrealistic to expect this for all double arm amputees and compromises have to be made. Some of these will only be temporary but others will be permanent. It is therefore important to establish early on in training those aspects of life for which independence is of prime importance and those areas in which the amputee is prepared to accept help or a lower level of achievement. These will vary with each individual and will depend partly on his personality and partly on his situation in life. They will vary according to his age, sex, marital status, nationality, occupation and hobbies. They will change during his life, for help which is acceptable in one situation becomes embarrassing in another. A married man with young children may feel that independence in dressing is less important than being able to earn a living to support his wife and family, while a widower whose family have grown up may have different priorities. A young unmarried man or woman will probably be more concerned with appearance than an older more settled person. A man accustomed to earning his living by the skill of his hands will be more worried about whether he will be able to work than the executive who has clerical assistance and relies on his personality, training and mental skills for success in his occupation. Discussion between the therapist and amputee is vital to establish what the short-term goals are to be even when complete independence is the ultimate goal.

A minimum of four weeks full-time training, approximately 120 hours, is necessary to teach a bilateral below-elbow amputee sufficient control and skill to tackle most activities of daily living. If one or both arms are amputated above the elbow proportionally longer initial training will be necessary. A period of consolidation and practice at home should then be beneficial, with a further session of training later. By this time the amputee will have discovered the areas in which he still needs help and this training period can take the form of problem-solving. Consideration of job prospects and further training should be discussed before the end of the initial training period to allow time for arrangements to be made. There will then be the minimum of time-lag between final completion of training and the beginning of employment or job training. The second period of training provides an excellent opportunity for assessment and practice in real life or simulated work situations.

SUGGESTED ACTIVITIES FOR PRACTICE

Practice is the key to successful use of arm prostheses. Most single arm amputees never practise enough with their prostheses because they have a sound hand to do three-quarters of the work. The double arm amputee is dependent on his prostheses and so he will have the incentive to practise until he is proficient. Even so it can be very boring for him in the early stages when activities have to be very simple and limited. Games have the advantage here over crafts for they can be broken down into simple repetitive movements and yet interest can be maintained by the variety and degree of complexity. The range of games is enormous and with minimal modifications of size and shape of counters and dice almost any board game can be used. The old favourites such as Solitaire, draughts, chess, Monopoly and Ludo, as well as the newer games such as Mastermind, Scrabble and war games, are all suitable. Cards, too, are excellent, though the bilateral arm amputee will need to use a card holder. This can be either a board made

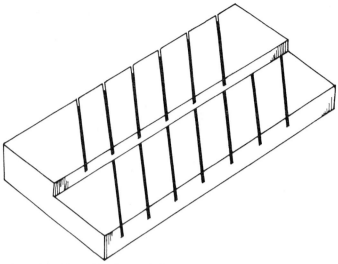

Fig. 39. A card-holder with diagonal slots.

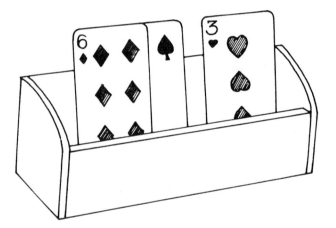

Fig. 40. A letter-rack type of card-holder.

with diagonal slots (Fig. 39) into which the cards have to be placed individually or a letter rack (Fig. 40) in which they can be placed as a pack and then spread out. The side of a lidded box placed upside down, so that the cards can be inserted between the lid and the box, makes a satisfactory substitute for a special holder. The advantages of card games over board games are that more people are familiar with them and play them at home; they can also be used equally effectively by single and double arm amputees as a training medium and so provide a good group activity.

Writing and typing

This is an essential part of the double arm amputee's training. Valuable practice in learning control for writing can be had from painting. At first this should be with a large brush, progressing to more controlled work with a smaller brush. The non-artistic may enjoy painting furniture and later painting by numbers, while the artistic can be encouraged to develop painting as a hobby. Typing should be done with each arm used for its respective side of the keyboard. Selected exercises from a typing book will be helpful as the typist will gradually learn the position of the keys by concentrating on words with a limited number of letters at one time. If the points of the hook tend to skid on the typewriter keys a rubber thimble or a small piece of rubber tubing held in the split hook and over one of the fingers should overcome this. For the first few typing sessions the paper should be put into the typewriter for the amputee, but he should be encouraged to do this for himself as soon as he has learnt to open and close his split hook at a specific point in space. He should first pull forward the paper release lever so that he can remove the old piece of paper, then insert a new sheet before pushing back this lever. He should then be able to wind in the new sheet by using the line space lever rather than trying to turn the roller knob. Once the paper is in the machine he can pull forward the paper release lever to adjust the paper if it is not straight, finally pushing this lever back before starting to type.

Once the amputee has learnt the minimum of skill he should be encouraged to write or type letters. This not only gives more purpose to the activity but will increase his self-esteem, maintain links with family and friends, and give them opportunities to support and encourage him with their approval. It also gives additional practice in folding the letter, inserting it into the envelope, tearing off and fixing the stamp and posting the letter. The amputee who knows shorthand can combine prosthetic training with vocational rehabilitation by taking down simple letters, typing, folding and then mailing them. This final stage provides an opportunity for using split hooks in public outside the hospital for posting the letter and buying stamps in the post office.

SIMPLE ACTIVITIES OF DAILY LIVING

These should be introduced into the programme as soon as possible. Activities which will help the amputee and allow him to help others will assist him in overcoming the feeling of dependence and use-lessness which is a marked feature of losing both hands. Playing a game with a child gives both of them practice with their prostheses and frees the therapist to treat another patient. Other activities of this kind can include: learning to handle the telephone and later being able to answer it and write down messages; doing errands for other patients and staff, particularly fetching and delivering things; learning to handle money, first on a table and then standing at a shop counter or sitting as in a bus; opening and closing doors with knobs, lever handles, bolts, Yale and mortice locks (lever handles are much the easiest to operate, oval knobs are possible but round knobs are extremely difficult and sometimes impossible to turn); plugging in and switching on lights, radio and television; opening and closing different types of windows; helping to make coffee and tea, including the washing up. By practising these skills in the sheltered environment of the occupational therapy department the amputee will have the opportunity to try out his skills without anxious stares from the curious as to how he will manage and with the advice of the therapist as to how best to tackle each activity. To begin with he will need quite a lot of help in positioning his prostheses and split hooks at the best angles and advice on how best to grasp an object or tool, but gradually he will learn to work this out for himself and the therapist should be able to withdraw her assistance gradually as the amputee gains in confidence.

FURTHER ACTIVITIES OF DAILY LIVING

Becoming independent for dressing and personal hygiene is probably one of the most difficult things that a double arm amputee has to learn. Some feel that it is not worth the effort involved to dress themselves routinely, but most agree that it is of value to learn how to be completely independent; one can then be selective about when and what one does for oneself. To know that one is able to be independent is more important than being independent all the time.

Toilet independence

The first aim for dressing independence must be geared to toilet independence. Men will need to have trousers with a zip in the fly and may need a small split-ring or loop of lace inserted in the tab to give a firm point of grasp for the split hook. Underpants of boxer style are easier than Y-fronts. Trousers should be loose fitting so that it is easy to operate the zip. A flat hook is easier to fasten than a press-stud at the waist but best of all is to have the zip extending to the top of the waistband with a tab fastened over it with a piece of Velcro. The double below-elbow amputee should have no difficulty getting his trousers and underpants up and down and most amputees find it easiest to use the cable lever for this purpose. The bilateral above-elbow amputee will have more difficulty. Some find it best to wear trousers with braces and have their underpants buttoned inside their trousers.

Women should wear pants of a slippery jersey-type material rather than stretch crêpe or elasticated material. Tights should be avoided in the early days of learning toilet independence so it is probably easiest to wear trousers rather than a skirt. These should have either an elasticated waist or a front zip fastening modified as for men's trousers. If a T-shirt or cosy top is worn there will be no additional problem of tucking in a vest smoothly.

The bilateral arm amputee with one below-elbow prosthesis should be able to manage toilet paper in his split hook. Soft tissue on a roll is easier to manage than the harder slippery toilet paper or that which is interleaved. A length of four or five pieces should be torn off the roll and wound round the tips of the split hook. If the amputee is unable to reach to cleanse himself from the back he should be able to reach from the front.

For the bilateral arm amputee unable to manage this method there are other alternatives:

1. A two-pronged toilet appliance mounted on a handle which fits into the chuck at the base of the split hook. This gives extra length and can be angled if necessary to make it more efficient. It can be carried in a knitting bag with a zip top when going out.

2. Position the toilet paper on the rim of the lavatory bowl or on the heel for cleansing (see Chapter 17).

3. Have a toilet appliance fitted on a swivel behind the lavatory so that it can be swung into position over the lavatory bowl for use. This has the disadvantage that it ties the person to using only the one lavatory.

4. A Clos-o-mat toilet which washes and dries on the press of a button is an expensive but very efficient solution for the severely disabled person. A cheaper alternative which some find satisfactory is to use a bidet.

Menstruation

A woman has the additional problem of coping with menstruation. She should be able to manage tampons if she has one below–elbow prosthesis. If sanitary towels are used the ones with adhesive strips at the back, which can be used inside ordinary panties, are probably the easiest to manage though some people prefer the towels which fasten in the front of the pantie. A close-fitting pantie must be worn and is sometimes difficult for the amputee to manage at first. Soluble towels which can be flushed down the lavatory do away with the task of wrapping for disposal.

Dressing

It is sometimes easier for the double arm amputee to put on garments when without prostheses as these easily become caught up in the material but this largely depends on the length of the stumps. The bilateral below–elbow amputee can probably completely dress himself without his prostheses except for fastenings, while the bilateral above-elbow amputee will be able to do little beyond putting on a T-shirt without his prostheses to help him. The point at which the prostheses are put on must be decided for each individual. This does not, of course, apply to those born without arms as they develop foot and mouth skills which are beyond the agility of the adult who loses both hands. Choice of clothes which are easy to manage can determine whether independence for dressing is going to be possible.

Clothing

Points to look for in selecting the most suitable clothes include:

1. Loose-fitting clothes with the minimum of fastenings, i.e. sweaters, T-shirts, jersey dresses, elasticated waists in skirts and slacks.
2. Sufficient room across the back of the garment to allow for the free use of the operating cords.
3. Loose-fitting sleeves and arm-holes. These do not restrict the operating cord and wear longer. Raglan sleeves for outer garments are ideal.
4. Underwear made of natural fibres should be worn under the prostheses and appendages to allow for the absorption of perspiration.
5. Men's underpants with straight front openings are easier than Y-fronts for learning toilet independence.
6. Slip-on shoes or boots with zip fastenings are easier than laced shoes, which will have to be modified with either elastic laces or fastened from top to bottom (see Fig. 33).
7. Velcro is a very simple fastening but is unsatisfactory on woollen materials, particularly knitted garments. When used the hook side should always face away from the skin and the pull be along the length of the Velcro not from selvedge to selvedge (see Fig. 6).

8. Metal zips are less likely to jam than coiled nylon ones.
9. Flat trouser hooks are easier to fasten at the waist than press-studs.
10. Brassières should have elastic shoulder straps for both comfort under the prostheses and so that they can be fastened in front and then turned to the back. Most bilateral arm amputees will need to have their bras modified with a pull-back fastening and a tape loop for tightening with their stump (Fig. 41).

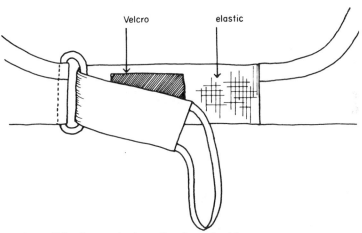

Fig. 41. A modification to the brassière for a double-arm amputee.

11. If stockings and a belt are worn the suspenders should be fastened prior to putting on. The belt and stockings can then be put on as one garment. The belt should have a zip, pull-back buckles or a pull-back Velcro fastening, not hooks.
12. Fine tights and stockings are difficult to put on without tearing. Fancy thicker ones are more practical for everyday wear if trousers are not acceptable. Tights which are open in the crutch can be worn with pants on top so that the tights do not have to be pulled down for going to the lavatory.
13. Buttonholes should be big enough for the button to slip through easily. Large coat buttons may be fastened with the split hooks, but for smaller buttons a button hook (see Fig. 76) will be necessary. This should be practised on a garment spread on the table before attempting it on oneself (p. 84).
14. Braces are often easier to manage than a tight-fitting waist fastening, particularly if both amputations are above-elbow.
15. Cuffs should be fastened with either expanding cuff-links or buttons on elastic thread so that the cuffs can be fastened before

putting on the shirt. Length of sleeves is important: if too long they will impede the function of the split hooks and if too short they will show more of the prosthesis than necessary. They should just cover the wrist rotary when the elbow is flexed to 90°.

16. Tying a tie is possible but tedious (p. 83). If clip-on ties or a tie-on elastic is acceptable it will be much easier to manage. With the tie on elastic it is not necessary to fasten the top button of the shirt.

17. Sports shirts which can be worn outside the trousers are easier to manage than the type with tails that need tucking in. If the latter are worn it may be necessary to cut off the back tail just below the waist and insert a piece of elastic to hold the back of the shirt snugly at waist level. Then only the front of the shirt has to be tucked into the trousers.

18. Anoraks with double zip fasteners should be avoided.

19. A self-winding wrist watch can be left permanently strapped to the prosthesis. Otherwise it may be necessary to wind the watch with the lips.

20. Women should choose brooches that can be pinned on before putting on the garment and necklaces that can be put on over the head ready fastened. Ears should be pierced if ear-rings are to be put on by the amputee.

21. Spectacles should be stable enough so that the arms stay open while being put on. The easiest way is to lay them open on a bed or a cushion and then put the head into the glasses.

Washing, shaving and cosmetics

Bathing has already been dealt with (p. 16) as it is of necessity done without the prostheses. Washing the face can be done with the prostheses on but is not advised because of the risk of getting water in the wrist mechanism. However, it is necessary to wash the split hooks regularly. A nailbrush that can be gripped firmly in the opposite split hook should be used and care taken to see that the gripping surface is clean and free from grease.

Shaving is probably best done as already described, using an electric razor on a stand (Fig. 12), although it is possible to use an electric razor with a below-elbow prosthesis.

Putting on cosmetics is largely dependent on a choice of holders that are easy to handle. Eye make-up should be in stick or pencil form. Creams and liquid make-up should be avoided. A solid powder combined with a base which can be applied with a piece of sheepskin is a good choice. Lipstick should be kept wound up and open on the dressing table as this is a tedious operation.

Use of cutlery

Before attempting to use a knife and fork together the bilateral arm amputee should learn how to pick up spoon, fork and knife individually. To pick up a spoon or fork the opposite hook should be placed on to the bowl of the spoon or prongs of the fork so that the handle lifts off the table. It can then be grasped easily. If the angle is not quite correct this can be adjusted while holding the spoon or fork in the mouth. If the fork is to be used for eating as well as holding the food steady for cutting it is better to use it with the prongs facing upwards. If the amputee decides to cut up the food first and then eat, it can be used prongs down for cutting and then turned around for eating. Most arm amputees cannot get the tip of the fork to the mouth if the prongs are facing down. The method decided on will depend on the individual's preference and the level of amputation. Bilateral below–elbow amputees can use either method efficiently, but the amputee with one arm off above the elbow may prefer both to cut his food and to eat with the below–elbow arm. He will therefore have to use the American method of eating.

The best way to pick up a knife and fork is to first pick up the fork as already described. Then pick up the blade of the knife between the tips of the other split hook and flip the handle over the operating cord lever with the fork, so that it rests against this lever when pressure is exerted for cutting (as for a pencil, see Fig. 29).

Picking up and drinking from a cup and a glass should now be tackled. The key to picking up a cup is to hold the bottom of the handle close to the bowl of the cup so that the weight of the cup rests on the

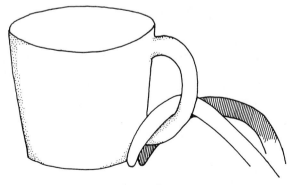

Fig. 42. Holding a cup in the split hook.

111

rigid finger of the split hook (Fig. 42). The shapes of cups and handles vary so it is worth practising with a variety to find the easiest. The size of glass that can be picked up will be dependent on the width of opening of the split hook. Many bilateral arm amputees find a wine glass gripped around the stem easier to manage than a tumbler.

Many amputees find it difficult at first to pick up sandwiches, bread and cakes with their split hooks. A holder made from rigid plastic material that can be moulded with heat will disperse the force of the split hook over a wider area (Fig. 43). Some people prefer to use a fork when eating soft easily crumbled foods, while others learn in time to maintain some tension on the operating cord to prevent complete closure of the split hook.

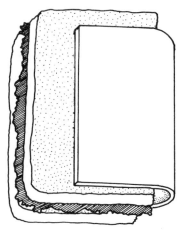

Fig. 43. A sandwich holder.

Hobbies and other interests

Skills practised by the bilateral arm amputee should not be limited to activities of daily living even though much time must be spent on these. The amputee's hobbies and interests should be studied to discover how best he can continue with them. Sometimes a related hobby can be started if the old one demanded more manual dexterity than the amputee now has. Modifications can often be made to equipment such as cameras and cars. An introduction can be made to a disabled sports association where the bilateral amputee can often contribute as well as compete, being more mobile than many of the other members.

Driving a car may be a necessity as well as a hobby. Although the double arm amputee should be discouraged from attempting to drive too soon after losing his hands, he should be reassured that he will be able to drive again. It is possible to drive a car with gears but most bilateral arm amputees find it easier to drive an automatic. Some like one or more knobs on the steering wheel while others prefer nothing. This is an individual choice and will depend on the person's level of amputation, skill with his prostheses and the type of car. Every arm amputee, whether he has lost one or both hands, will need to re-take the driving test. He will be tested on his ability to control the car and not on the modifications and aids he has in the car. Before starting to drive the double arm amputee should consider the following points:

1. Can he control the steering wheel with both arms equally well or with one arm more easily?

2. If he can only use one arm efficiently to control the steering wheel will he be able to (a) change gear with the other arm or (b) steady the wheel with the other prosthesis while changing gear?

3. Can he manage the handbrake of all makes of cars with either arm or only certain types or with only one arm?

4. Can he reach and work the indicators, lights, dip switch, windscreen wipers and horn without losing control of the car or taking his eyes off the road?

The answers to these questions will determine whether he should drive with prostheses, what sort or car he should choose and whether he will need to have further modifications made to a standard car before he can safely drive it.

Success at a hobby will depend on the determination of the amputee, but it is known that many do continue a wide range of interests including carpentry, home decorating, embroidery, gardening and art. Others find that their job leaves little energy for an active hobby and prefer to pursue a less physically demanding interest such as spectator sports, listening to music and walking.

Job evaluation

If a person who has lost both hands wants to return to his former job every effort should be made to discover whether this is possible. Most employers have very little idea of the capabilities of a person with two arm prostheses. It is therefore essential that someone who knows the amputee's potential visits the employer to discover exactly what his former job entailed. Ideally this should be the occupational therapist responsible for the training of the amputee but sometimes it is more politic for the first approach to be made by the Disablement Resettlement Officer or social worker. If the work seems suitable and the employer is prepared to cooperate, a full job evaluation should be made. The amputee can then be assessed within the hospital or rehabilitation unit as to his capability of carrying out the work in the time allowed. Sometimes specific pieces of equipment can be borrowed or similar ones found within the hospital so that the amputee can practise until he is confident. The technical officer may need to be drawn into the team if equipment needs to be modified or special tools made.

Before he starts work a visit should be made by the occupational therapist with the amputee to check that not only can he do his job satisfactorily but also that he is able to cope with the other facilities within the building. For example, can he manage all the door handles which he will need to use? If he needs to use a lift, is this possible? Will he be able to manage unaided in the canteen and the cloakroom? How is he going to travel to and from work? If a machine has had to be modified the technician should come also to check that the amputee can now work it safely and efficiently. If he is to work at a desk is it at the best height and are telephones, filing cabinets, etc. positioned for easy use? Often a minor rearrangement of furniture or the changing of the type of door handle makes all the difference between a double arm amputee managing a job efficiently and failing. Lastly, but perhaps the most important, this visit gives an opportunity for the employers and other employees to meet and see that a person with two artificial arms has the skills necessary for his job. With the therapist there the amputee should have confidence that he will get help and advice if necessary and the employers will know that there is someone that they can contact if a particular skill within the amputee's work becomes a problem in the future.

Some amputees will not want to return to their former job, particularly if the accident happened at work. They may prefer to take the opportunity of a new career with training at a Skills Centre, a university or a technical college. Alternatively they may wish to try and find a job in the open market with the skills that they already have. In the United Kingdom the DRO should be able to help bridge the gap between hospital and training course or work. A DP2 form should be completed for the amputee so that the DRO can play his part in the resettlement of the amputee. However, it should be stressed that the double arm amputee without either training or experience will find it very difficult to find employment in the open market. The therapist should study his aptitudes and give him as much opportunity as possible to try out different work situations, concentrating on those exploiting his potential abilities of personality, experience, mobility, language and other mental skills. In some occupations bilateral arm amputees have already proved their ability. These include PBX telephone switchboard operators, a variety of clerical jobs, artists and draughtsmen, executive and legal occupations and teachers. But there are a growing number of other occupations open to them as skilled manual jobs become increasingly computer-operated. Care should be taken that the amputee with skills that qualify him for a satisfying job does not finish up as a lift operator or a car-park attendant because potential employers are unaware of his capabilities.

Home visits

As well as visiting the amputee's prospective place of work the occupational therapist should visit his home. It is here that he is going to tackle many of the more difficult skills including dressing and bathing. If the double arm amputee is a woman who is returning to run her own home, it is also her place of work and must be viewed as such.

A home visit also gives the therapist the opportunity to meet more of the family and friends. Presumably she will have already talked to the immediate family about how they can help the amputee achieve independence, but she may not have had a chance to meet all the children, the extended family and some of the closer friends. They are all probably anxious to help and certainly curious to know how the amputee is going to manage so many things. They are naturally nervous of relying on him for skilled tasks. For the amputee this can be very frustrating when his confidence in his own ability has been built up within the hospital. A quiet reassuring word that he can manage, and must be allowed to try even if he fails at first, may help to smooth the transition from hospital to home. There are also practical problems to investigate. Door handles should be levers or the doors have a spring catch. Locks on front and back doors should be checked to make sure that they can be operated. Can he reach and turn bath, basin and sink taps both with and without prostheses? Can he reach the toilet paper easily when sitting on the lavatory? Can he manage the controls on the radio and television? Is there a hook in the bathroom to hang his towel on when drying his back? Is there a suitable chair to hang his prostheses over when putting them on? Is the kitchen or dining table a convenient height for eating? Can he operate the cooker taps or knobs and the switch for the electric kettle? Whether these latter are to be modified or not will depend on how much the amputee plans to do in the kitchen; for the man living on his own or a woman running her home it is essential that they are easily operated. In the United Kingdom the Gas and Electricity Boards are very helpful about changing taps and switches for any handicapped person. For anyone working in the kitchen with two artificial arms certain features will make life easier:

1. A continuous flat surface between cooker and work top so that pans can be slid off the cooker without lifting.
2. An oven with shelves that can be pulled out safely so that casseroles can be stirred or inspected without having to lift them from the oven. A cooker with shelves on the door is ideal.
3. A plate rack eliminates drying of crockery and reduces breakages.
4. Narrow shelves so that tins and jars are stored 'one deep'.
5. Hooks for cups or half-shelves so that china can be reached easily.
6. A trolley with easy-running castors combined with a level floor between kitchen and dining area is easier, safer and less tiring than repeated journeys with a tray.
7. A clean milk bottle kept by the sink for filling kettle and saucepans in situ.
8. A patient family who do not mind waiting for meals and helping with the washing up!

Another skill that the housewife will need to master is washing and ironing. An automatic washing machine is a great help, particularly if it tumble-dries as well as washes. If there is no washing machine available it is probably worth taking the weekly wash to a laundrette. The amputee should at least get a spin drier for wringing clothes with bilateral arm prostheses it is not only difficult but very tedious. Ironing is less tiring with a lightweight iron but some are easier to handle than others; the amputee should try several makes before deciding which one to get if her own is unsatisfactory. There are many other labour-saving gadgets for use in the home which will make the bilateral arm amputee's life easier.

Many things must be considered in the home and probably only the essentials can be looked at on the first visit. However, once the idea of modifying the environment to suit a person's capabilities has been sown, most families will be able to do much of the planning on their own. The solutions worked out by the double arm amputee and his family are much more likely to work than any arrangement imposed on them from outside.

CHAPTER 14

The Arm Amputee with an Additional Disability

When more than one disability exists it is essential to draw up a programme of priorities. Many patients cannot tolerate treatment in several areas at once and yet they need to be reassured that all aspects of their disability will be covered. The doctor in charge of the patient's treatment will decide when to start treatment of each disability. The therapists in charge of the different treatment areas must then work together to plan a realistic and balanced programme. If they continue to work closely they will find that many areas of personal independence are best tackled as a joint project.

Triple and quadruple amputees

When one arm and both legs are amputated the patient usually receives training first in the use of his leg prostheses, progressing to arm training once he has developed balance on his lower limb prostheses. The exception to this is when the patient is elderly and has little prospect of learning to walk on his lower limbs. If both arms and one leg have been lost it is essential to start training earlier in the use of upper limb prostheses. The amputee will be equally well motivated to walk and to learn to use his artificial arms so a shared programme should be practical.

When both arms and both legs are involved the decision about which area to start on will depend on the age and the prognosis of the patient. Many elderly quadruple amputees have a better prospect of learning some independence with their arm prostheses than they have with their lower limbs. However, the desire to walk is very strong and many quadruple amputees will not believe at this early stage that they have a better prospect of independence in a wheelchair than on lower limb prostheses.

For triple and quadruple amputees who can walk and yet need a

117

stick, one can be fitted with an adaptor so that it slots directly into the arm prosthesis. This provides a stable walking aid and in the case of the triple amputee with one sound arm leaves that hand free for carrying objects, opening doors, etc. The quadruple amputee may need two such sticks for walking, but if so he will be considerably handicapped in having no means of doing anything else with his arm prostheses without removing at least one stick.

Many triple and quadruple amputees are elderly, losing their limbs because of cardiovascular insufficiency. To aim for complete independence is unrealistic. Far better to set short-term goals which will improve the quality of their life and perhaps give a measure of independence within a sheltered environment. The elderly lady with both legs and one hand missing will get far more satisfaction from being able to knit for her grandchildren and help prepare the vegetables than from struggling for complete independence in dressing and bathing, for which community services can be used. Few elderly people with this degree of handicap will be able to live alone and so it is more important that they adjust to their disability and find ways to live a contented life than to be constantly striving to overcome a severe handicap.

The young triple amputee who loses his limbs as the result of an accident is a different proposition. He should be encouraged to aim for complete personal independence and return to work. Much support will be needed to achieve this goal, with maximum use being made of facilities to modify the home and place of work. Use should be made of self-help equipment such as hoists, lifts and modified self-drive vehicles. For the severely handicapped person who has the ability and genuine desire to return to work there is a wealth of good-will within the community to help overcome what might seem to be insurmountable problems.

Hemiplegic single arm amputees

Occasionally a single arm amputee has the misfortune to lose the use of his only sound hand as the result of a stroke and he may have associated speech, communication and perception problems. If the paralysis is severe he will need to learn to use his prosthesis for dominant arm activities and his training in the use of the prosthesis will proceed much as for a double arm amputee. At the same time he may be having speech therapy and physiotherapy so a team approach is essential if the patient is not to become confused.

If the amputation is very high the patient may find it easier to feed himself with his paralysed arm. To do this he may need a ball-bearing arm support and a self-righting spoon. This is a very individual problem where the residual abilities must be carefully assessed so that the maximum use can be made of them. One man in his early forties suffered such an accident and subsequently returned to his former job after just over a year's rehabilitation. To achieve such a result demanded cooperation from employers and family with modifications not only to the equipment to be used but also to hours of work. This man decided that returning to work was more important to him than complete personal independence and so concentrated his effort on this area of his life. Another person with a similar handicap but different responsibilities might choose a different course.

Blind arm amputees

Usually blindness associated with amputation is the result of an accident. Often both arms are affected, but, as the blind person relies on touch to compensate for his lost sight, he should be fitted with only one prosthesis. This should be on the dominant side unless this stump is markedly longer than the other. A cosmetic prosthesis which can be secured with the minimum of straps should be available for the other stump.

The blind amputee should be encouraged to handle his prosthesis and terminal device before it is first put on, so that he can develop a mental picture of its components. Similarly at each stage of training time should be allowed for him to feel the position of the split hook and the degree of opening. The above-elbow amputee should also feel the angle of the elbow and the position of the split hook in relation to his body. In this way he will gradually build up a picture of the operation of the prosthesis and terminal device, by associating it with the weight of the prosthesis on his stump, the tension of the operating cord and the degree of movement required to achieve the desired result.

With one hand or stump free to feel with, the blind amputee learns to identify objects and then to pick them up with his prosthesis. He progresses to learning to manipulate them within his split hook, for example positioning a pencil or spoon in the split hook.

Practice in self-feeding should be started with a biscuit or piece of toast held in the split hook, progressing to using first a spoon and then a fork. Picking up a cup should be practised with an empty cup until the amputee has mastered the pattern of shoulder and elbow movement necessary to keep the cup level while taking it up to his mouth.

Paper for writing should be clamped under two horizontal strips of wood to act as a guide to size and direction. These should be kept at least 2.5 cm (1 in) apart in the early stages. Typing will probably provide a more realistic means of communication. A cover for the keyboard with holes above the keys will be necessary. It is a help if the blind amputee can memorize the order of the keys before starting to type, otherwise he should start with only a limited number of keys available for use.

Practice in using a telephone may open up a possible employment prospect. At least one blind double arm amputee operates a modified PBX telephone switchboard (Fig. 36). Time spent in encouraging the blind amputee to recognize sounds and to remember names and messages will help him in his future search for employment.

The top of the standard white stick can be easily modified with a short piece of dowel shaped to fit snugly into the chuck at the base of the split hook while being held between the 'fingers'. The stick then becomes an extension of the prosthesis and can be used as an aid to walking.

Close cooperation with the Royal National Institute for the Blind, or St Dunstans in the case of a serviceman, is necessary to make sure that training with the prosthesis is coordinated with their 'sight' training in independence.

Other additional handicaps

It is, of course, possible to have any handicap in addition to amputation. Usually these do not affect the ability to operate the split hook and the prosthesis but influence the use which can be made of it. A heart condition, limiting the amount of effort allowed, or restricted movement of the back, affecting balance, are two obvious examples. An additional handicap of this type will influence the choice of activities and the goals set, but will not demand a change in fitting and training procedure.

An additional handicap which prevents the normal operation and control of the prosthesis and split hook will need a different approach. An example of this is spasticity coupled with amputation which makes controlled movement of the limb difficult if not impossible. Two possible methods of giving such an amputee some use of his prosthesis are either by linking his prosthesis to an arm support or by giving him external power to control the split hook. The choice will depend on whether the aim is to control the prosthesis in space, as for feeding or writing, or to control the grasp mechanism of the split hook or wrist rotation for pre-positioning the split hook.

To link a ball-bearing arm support to a prosthesis, the hinged pivot which is normally screwed to the underside of the forearm support is

120

riveted to the underneath of the prosthetic forearm. In order to decide on the best position for this pivot it is advisable initially to strap the prosthesis to the forearm support. With this support the spastic amputee can often learn to feed himself, use an electric typewriter, turn pages of a book and paint.

The spastic amputee who has some control of his arm in space but is unable to combine this with operation of the split hook might benefit from having an externally powered split hook controlled by another part of the body. This can give independent prehension for activities such as manipulating a tape recorder, switching on a radio or television, picking up a pen and a spoon. One such amputee with a high level amputation on one side, severe spasticity in the other arm and confined to a wheelchair controlled his split hook from switches fixed to the arm of his wheelchair.

Complete independence is not realistic for these amputees but if the quality of their life can be improved they will become happier people who can contribute something to the society in which they live.

PART IV

Limb–deficient Children and Child Arm
Amputees

CHAPTER 15

Prosthesis, Appliance or Nothing?

It is normal to feel that a child born with all or part of a limb missing should have an artificial replacement for that limb. Society has conditioned us to want to look the same as everyone else. We assume that this child will feel likewise. Exposed to the same pressures to accept these norms he probably will want to conform but he may not be prepared to accept the penalties that such compliance imposes. We are born with two arms and two legs and as we grow up these become part of our body image. To lose part of our body is a tragedy to us. We mourn our loss and long for the return of the limb or at least some sort of artificial replacement which we think will make us look more normal and make it possible to achieve some of those goals which we feel will now be impossible. But if we are born without a part of the body we never build that part into the image that we have of ourself and so cannot miss in the same way what we have never had. As the child matures he realizes that he is different. He may develop a need for a prosthesis to complete his body in response to the community in which he lives. He is unlikely to feel the need for an arm prosthesis for practical achievement until he is too old to adjust to its disadvantages. We, the adults concerned with the child's present and future mental and physical health, must therefore decide for him whether the advantages of early fitting and training with one or more prostheses, outweigh the disadvantages.

Successful wearing of prostheses by young children appears to be governed by two factors. The prosthesis must increase the range of activities available to the child and they must be cost-effective in terms of effort. Appearance does not play an appreciable part in the acceptance or rejection of prostheses by very young children. Repeatedly very young children are successfully fitted with prostheses which fulfil a need of the child at that time. But children's needs change and once prostheses no longer satisfy the current need they will cease to be cost-effective and be discarded. The child with one prosthesis is more tolerant of its shortcomings because he is less dependent on it. If it does not help him he just ignores it and does not use it. The child with two or more prostheses will not tolerate wearing prostheses that restrict his function. If he is not allowed to discard them he will show his frustration by psychological disturbance.

A prosthesis will only be cost-effective to a child if it is easy to operate with the minimum of practice, and not liable to frequent breakdowns. To the best of my knowledge this hypothesis has never been fully tested or proven but it is supported by observations, records of acceptance and rejection of prostheses and the comments of older children. A conventional non-powered prosthesis is only cost-effective if the wearer has an efficient lever to control and operate it, while an externally powered prosthesis (at the moment limited to upper limbs) seems to need to become progressively more sophisticated as the child's needs develop. Control of the prosthesis in space and position servo, which are an integral part of the EPP (extended physiological proprioception) arm prosthesis developed in Edinburgh, do seem to be particularly pertinent to the value of prostheses to the child with bilateral amelia of the upper limbs.

It is generally accepted that children will tolerate lower limb prostheses at an earlier age and with less formal training than they will accept upper limbs when two or more limbs are effected. This is despite the fact that the normal child learns to manipulate objects with his hands before he starts to walk. The child's first lower limb prostheses are simple to operate and though they may require a considerable amount of effort, very little finesse is needed to control them. The child is highly motivated to walk when first fitted and the protheses makes fulfilment of this need possible. As the child grows older this motivation weakens and the importance of stable levers to control the prostheses becomes more evident. Unless these are present most children without good upper limbs to assist them with walking eventually reject lower limb prostheses. Four-limb deficient children without either stable hip or shoulder joints find it easier to move around on the floor or, as they get older, in an electric chair. Lower limb prostheses are no longer cost-effective for them. Children with stable hip joints plus reasonable length levers to control the prostheses can and do make efficient use of lower limb prostheses. If their arms are severely shortened they will find it much more difficult to balance and may have to be content with shorter than average lower limbs. Children with only one leg affected should have no difficulty in learning to walk and also to run if they have a strong lever of reasonable length.

126

Parental acceptance of limb deficiency

The attitudes of the parents towards their child and his handicap is of prime importance. Their approval or disapproval, acceptance or rejection, and feelings about the limb deficiency or loss will determine how the child feels about it. Wilma Gurney (1958), the Senior Medical Social Worker in the Child Amputee Project at the University of California, found that parents applying to the project for help fell into three main groups:

1. Those that had adjusted to having given birth to a child with an anomaly sufficiently well to be able to discuss the handicap realistically. They had accepted that the child needed to be both independent and dependent and had been able to free themselves sufficiently from self-blame to be able to communicate understanding to the child and try to help him with his problems of being different from other children.

2. Parents who were still bewildered and felt responsible for the child's handicap; who were easily upset by the reaction of relatives, friends and strangers to their child's anomaly and to the idea of a prosthesis, but yet who appreciated that they and their child needed help.

3. Those parents who had been unable to accept their child's handicap and had absorbed the child into their own needs and conflicts. They tended to isolate themselves and insist that they were self-sufficient.

She found that the majority of parents fell into the second group, and felt that most of them needed considerable help themselves before they were able to help their child accept and make use of a prosthesis. It is natural to feel upset and sorry for any child who has a handicap. To let that pity overwhelm one's good sense can harm the child rather than help him. Sometimes it is worth questioning whether one is really sorry for the child or upset because one finds the situation distressing oneself. The limb-deficient child has the same needs as any other child. He needs to be loved and accepted unconditionally by his parents, to feel secure within the circle of his family so that he is able to see his handicap in perspective as one facet of himself and not the overriding influence. People are bound to react abnormally to what is unknown to them. First the parents and then the child must show them that they do not allow the limb deficiency to alter their behaviour. It may influence their lives but need not affect their relationships.

A child who loses a hand is in rather a different position. If he is still a baby he will quickly forget what it was like to have that limb, but the

127

young child who has started to use the limb will react violently to its loss. He will also react to his parents' behaviour at this time of stress. Their grief and feeling of responsibility will tend to make them try to compensate to the child. His distress and resentment at his loss will tend to make him reject the deficient limb. Over-compensation by his parents may lead him to realize that he can trade on his loss to achieve other previously unattainable goals. Either way he is not going to be very amenable to training in the use of his prosthesis although he will probably be quite keen to wear it. The older child, whose reason is beginning to overrule his emotions, will more quickly adjust to the idea of a useful prosthetic replacement, particularly if it is possible to find an important interest for which it is of positive value.

Types of limb deficiency

The most common type of congenital limb deficiency is to be born with one hand missing (87 such children were referred to the limb-fitting services in England in 1974, whereas only 20 children were referred with a leg missing). In the same year 7 children with both arms affected were referred and 6 with both legs involved. The types of deficiencies associated with thalidomide are extremely rare but do occur for no known reason. There are no separate figures for child traumatic amputees but from experience these are less common than congenital absences.

Some children are born with only part of the hand missing, some with all the fingers absent but with the base of the palm still present, others with a complete forearm but no remnant of a hand and most common of all are those born with a small remnant of forearm. All these deficiencies are known as transverse hemimelia. They look as if the limb has been amputated or rather as if it has just stopped growing. This term also applies to those absences which are through-elbow and above-elbow. A complete absence of the arm is termed amelia.

Other children have one or more fingers but a shortened arm. This can be a paraxial deficiency or a phocomelia. A paraxial deficiency is when the upper part of the limb is normal but only one-half of the forearm develops with either the ulnar or radial fingers. A phocomelia refers to a limb in which the proximal part is missing. This can range from just the head of the humerus to the whole arm and results in a deformity that varies from a single digit to a deformed hand and forearm attached at shoulder level. Although this type of deficiency often presents a functional hand it lacks stability and power because of the absence of a normal shoulder joint. Similar types of deficiencies occur in the lower limbs.

128

For its manipulative ability the hand relies on sensation and dexterity. Without sensation dexterity cannot exist, but with sensation one needs remarkably little dexterity to achieve a high degree of manipulative ability. The limb-deficient child has this sensation. He has the same precise sensation in the end of his incomplete arm as we have in the tips of our fingers. With this sensation he is able to achieve a remarkable degree of manipulative ability. This particularly applies to the child with a full length forearm which he can use easily in apposition to his other hand. This factor must not be forgotten when deciding whether a prosthesis will be a help or hindrance to a particular limb-deficient child.

Types of prostheses

PASSIVE MITTEN

A simple soft prosthesis can be fitted safely on a very young child with a unilateral hemimelia. It consists of a rigid socket extending to normal wrist length with a soft plastic foam-filled mitt covering it and is held in place with the minimum of ribbon appendages. This type of prosthesis is normally fitted as soon as the child has sitting balance so that he can start to develop a two-handed pattern of achievement and learn to crawl.

BELOW-ELBOW PROSTHESIS

Once the child is walking confidently he is usually ready for a prosthesis which will give him independent grasp. He is then fitted with a standard type of cable-controlled prosthesis with a wrist unit and a detachable hand so that a small split hook with pink plastic covers can be used. Sometimes this type of prosthesis is fitted before the child is mature enough to learn to operate it himself so that he can begin to learn that his prosthesis is capable of holding and carrying objects. In this case the operating cord may be omitted until the mother and therapist report that the child is beginning to show interest in opening the split hook with his other hand. This pattern of fitting is now universally accepted and is supported by research carried out in various centres (Syphiewski 1972). Some below-elbow prostheses require a cup socket and occasionally a Munster type fitting (p. 33) because of the shortness of the forearm. Very young children often require a chest strap to keep the appendages on their shoulders. In the United Kingdom it is not standard practice to fit an above-elbow corset to a below-elbow prosthesis although in other countries this is a common practice.

Children with a paraxial type of deficiency can sometimes be fitted satisfactorily with a standard type of prosthesis. A window is cut in the socket to allow the finger to protrude outside for use when sensation is important. Despite this the combination of the restriction of use of a highly sensitive digit and the weak and often unstable lever provided by the deformed forearm often leads to rejection of this type of prosthesis. Similarly the child with a through-wrist or mid-palm deficiency often finds their own unformed arm more useful than this type of prosthesis.

ABOVE-ELBOW PROSTHESIS

The child without an elbow joint but with a sound shoulder joint and a reasonable length of humerus will be able to operate a cable-controlled above-elbow prosthesis. For the very young child this will have either a rigid or a friction elbow joint and can be supplied with a soft plastic mitten initially. A manually operated lock can be added to the friction joint if a positive lock is required before the child is old enough to learn to use a cable-controlled elbow lock. This is normally fitted when the child is approaching school age and is operated in the same way as the adult elbow lock (p. 68). The child with a long above-elbow stump or whose arm is absent from the elbow joint will need to have the lock positioned on an external side steel, which tends to make the upper arm bulky. Later the lock can usually be fitted internally as the shortened arm tends to develop at a slower pace than the normal limb.

THROUGH-SHOULDER PROSTHESIS

A child with complete absence of an arm (amelia) has no lever to control a prosthesis or with which to operate a conventional split hook. A phocomelia is an unstable lever with little power. It is for these children that externally powered prostheses may have something to offer. These prostheses are fitted on a jacket or enlarged shoulder cap, have either friction or powered shoulder and wrist joints, a powered split hook and either cable or powered elbow joint. In the United Kingdom carbon dioxide gas is used to provide the power and the movements are usually controlled by trunk movement, the phocomelic digits, the acromion process or stump movements. Initially the child is fitted with simple pat-a-cake prostheses controlled by flexion and extension of the body at waist level, with which he is able to pick up, hold and drop objects held between the prostheses. Later he is supplied with a powered split hook, then wrist rotation and finally a cable-controlled elbow or a linked powered shoulder, elbow and wrist. Age of fitting these various components will depend on the individual child's degree of disability, his development and the attitude of his parents. As a general rule a child with a bilateral arm deficiency and normal feet, which he can use for prehension, will not be interested in learning to use arm prostheses until he has standing balance and is wanting to walk, thus making his feet unavailable for grasp.

ALTERNATIVE APPLIANCES

Some children find the standard prosthesis irksome to wear and of little functional value in comparison to their ability without it. This is particularly true of the children with almost full length arms, those with no arms and those with either a paraxial deficiency or phocomelia.

The high degree of sensory discrimination present in the distal end of the congenitally shortened limb makes the wearing of any prosthesis irksome and could be likened to covering the hand with a

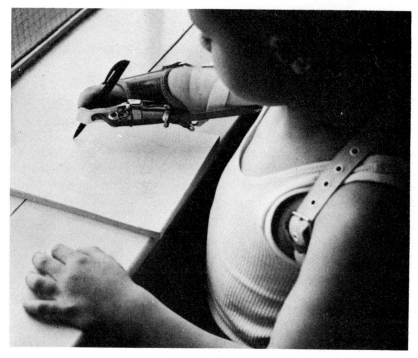

Fig. 44. A hinged opposition plate mounted on an open-ended socket gives both sensation and grasp.

boxing glove. For the child with a severely shortened arm the additional length plus the ability to grasp compensates to some extent for this loss. But for the child with a nearly full length arm the loss of sensation is more keenly felt. Attempts have been made at different centres to find a satisfactory prosthesis for these children by leaving the end of the socket open and off-setting the split hook or by fitting a hinged opposition plate controlled by the operating cord (Fig. 44). An alternative that is sometimes acceptable is to fit a lightweight rigid plastic opposition appliance that the child can slip on and off as it is needed (Fig. 45). Another possibility is for the child to have a wrist

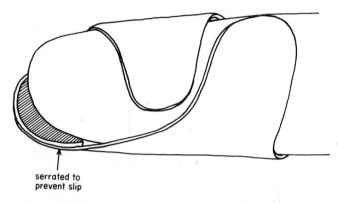

serrated to
prevent slip

Fig. 45. A plastic opposition plate suitable for a mid-palm deficiency.

strap into which he can insert the handle of tools for stability (see Fig. 48). Opposition appliances must be carefully moulded so that they do not cause pressure sores and must be readjusted at frequent intervals to keep pace with growth. Initially these appliances are often better made in the occupational therapy department where frequent remoulding during use is possible. Once the child knows what he wants of the appliance a more durable one can be made by the prosthetist.

HOOK OR HAND?

It is natural for parents to want their child to look as normal as possible. They will invariably opt for the prosthetic hand for their child unless they are convinced of the functional superiority of the split hook. The young child will only accept the split hook if his parents favour it. Why should the parents and child be persuaded to wear such an unnatural looking tool in place of a hand? The main reason is that it gives the child independent grasp with that arm. Attempts have been made to design a cosmetically acceptable functional hand which is lightweight and easy to operate. Up to now the hands that have been designed fall down on one or more of these criteria. The practice in the United Kingdom is to supply children, as adults, with a relatively non-functional but reasonably cosmetic hand which is detachable at the wrist so that a split hook can be used as required. The problem is then to decide when the child needs the split hook and when he is better off with a hand. Children, unlike adults, are using their arms all the time for exploring their environment and learning about objects. They should wear their split hooks routinely except for a purely social occasion when appearance becomes of prime importance, for example, being a bridesmaid, or perhaps a first visit to school before the other children have been told about the split hook.

The infant split hook normally supplied in the United Kingdom has pink plastic covers to try to make it more acceptable until the child and his parents have had a chance to learn its value. It is referred to as the child's 'fingers' and not as a split hook. Young children are not influenced by the appearance of their 'fingers' and are usually intrigued by its action. However, they will learn to consider it unacceptable if parents and close friends show distaste at its appearance. Ideally the young child should wear his 'fingers' all the time until he shows that he is disturbed by its appearance. This does not usually occur until puberty by which time he should be old enough to know when he needs his 'fingers' and when he can manage with the cosmetic hand.

Training

A child cannot be expected to use an arm prosthesis unless he is taught how to do so. Many people think that because a child needs little formal training to learn to walk with a leg prosthesis similarly he will learn automatically to use an arm prosthesis. Experience supported by research carried out by Wendt and Shaperman (1970) shows that this is not necessarily so. Only 4 of 17 children fitted but not trained in Los Angeles 'learnt' how to use their fingers. This is not surprising when one considers that we are asking the child to use a tool without the sensory stimulation to do so. A child feels the weight of his body on his stump as on the sole of his feet and is stimulated to walk by the desire to get to a specific place or object and by the encouragement of parents, siblings and other adults around him. To use his hand for grasp the child is stimulated by the feel of the object, but he has no tactile 'feel' in the fingers of his prosthetic hand or 'fingers'. He must be taught to open and close the 'fingers' and how to use them to complement his other hand. Even before this he must be taught to use this extension to his arm in conjunction with his other hand, for holding large objects and for supporting his weight when crawling. Training should therefore start as soon as he has his first prosthesis and not wait until he is ready to learn to use his 'fingers' for prehension.

Early training is in the form of advice to the parents about suitable activities to encourage the child to use his prosthesis and should not necessitate extra visits to the limb-fitting centre. Later when he gets his first working prosthesis more formal training will need to be started, with the mother continuing to take an active role in the child's training. How this is arranged will depend on the family's circumstances and the distance between home and the training centre. For the very young child a training session once a week or fortnight, with specific goals for the mother to work towards at home, provides sufficient guidance and stimulation to keep the programme going. If the gaps between visits are too long the mother tends to lose heart and the child loses interest, while treatment sessions closer together will not necessarily produce quicker results, for progress depends on the child's gradual maturing. An older child will tolerate a more concentrated period of training but even so requires time to practise what he has learnt in training in the natural environment of home. Once the child has reached the goal set for that period of training, visits should be discontinued until he is ready to progress to the next skill. Continuous training can be non-productive for child, parents and therapist. By the time he is to start school the child should have mastered the use of his prosthesis for all the activities that he is likely to meet there.

Further training may be necessary to learn specific skills at a later stage when short concentrated periods of training can be arranged to coincide with school holidays. A child who is a good prosthetic user will usually discover for himself how to tackle most new activities, needing only occasional advice and the opportunity to try out other appliances as his interests widen. The occupational therapist should always be available when the child visits the limb-fitting centre for routine checks, so that any small difficulty can be dealt with before it becomes a problem.

References

Gurney, W. (1958) Parents of children with congenital amputation. *Children*. Report of the US Department of Health, Education and Welfare.

Syphiewski, B. L. (1972) The child with terminal transverse hemimelia: A review of the literature on prosthetic management. *Artif. Limbs,16(1)*, 20–50.

Wendt, J. D. & Shaperman, J. (1970) The infant with a cable-controlled hook. *Am. J. occup. Ther., XXIV(6)*, 393–402.

CHAPTER 16

Growing Up with One Hand Missing

A very young child does not consider that having only one hand is in any way extraordinary. He will discover that he has only one hand and the rest of his family have two and he may remark on it or ask why, but he will not be upset by it. To him it is the same as some people being tall and others short, or some people having no hair or others wearing glasses. It is a difference but has no other significance to him. It is only when he discovers that other people think that it is odd that it begins to affect him. Then, if he is confident that it does not affect how his parents feel towards him, he will learn to accept it and gradually realize that he has a right to be different. There are bound to be traumatic occurrences when it is tempting to think that the absence of the hand is the cause, but usually it is not although it can aggravate the situation. It is just part of growing up, when constant adjustments have to be made to the demands of society. One of the ways adults concerned with the child's well-being can help him come to terms with his disability is to ensure that the handicap is only minimal.

Games to encourage two-handedness

The child who uses his limbs in a natural way is not noticed as being different, while the child who moves awkwardly, or tries to do bimanual activities with one hand only, attracts attention. The aim of fitting a prosthesis or appliance is not just to complete the body schema but also to help the child use his limbs in as normal a way as possible. If the prosthesis or appliance is found to be more of a hindrance than a help in fulfilling this aim the child should not be forced to wear it, but rather an alternative should be found that satisfies the child's needs at that particular time.

Games should be chosen that are suitable for the child's age and stage of development, remembering that a short period frequently

135

repeated is better than persevering with an activity after the child has lost interest. Specific activities should be slotted into normal play so that they are just part of the day and not a special training session. The aim is to encourage the child to use the prosthesis and shortened arm in a natural fashion and not as a party piece.

Games to encourage the use of both hands together include playing with any lightweight object that is too big to be picked up or carried in one hand such as large balls, balloons, teddy bears and dolls. At first the object should be given to the child, who will probably drop it. Later he should be encouraged to carry it short distances and finally to pick it up himself. The child can be encouraged to focus on the prosthesis as a useful tool by using it to knock down towers of bricks or to carry lightweight objects, such as a plastic bucket or bag looped over the hand into which he can put small toys.

He will need to build up strength in the arm ready for when he has an operating cord to open his 'fingers'. He should be encouraged to use the prosthesis for crawling and leaning on when playing on the floor. He will not be able to use it for grasp to pull himself up so parents should make a point of getting him to pull with that arm when he wants help in getting to his feet and in general rough-and-tumble play on the floor. They should sometimes hold that arm rather than his normal hand when walking, or if they feel insecure doing this make an opportunity for walking him between two adults so that both arms are held.

Grasp and release: learning more skill

Very young children are interested in dropping things before they want to pick them up. We have all seen the litter of toys around a baby's pram or cot with nothing left inside. This desire can be made use of when first teaching a young child to operate his 'fingers'. A bowl of water is placed on the floor just in front of the child and a small plastic animal or soldier is put into the child's 'fingers'. Very quickly the child realizes that if he reaches forward with his arm the 'fingers' open and the toy falls with a satisfying splash into the water. Most children enjoy this game, with the therapist or mother tiring of it long before they do. Gradually the child will realize that it is his pushing forward that opens the 'fingers' and will be able to respond to the request to open his 'fingers' if coupled with the therapist holding the object to be grasped just in front of the child. As he learns to control this operation the need for greater skill can be gradually inserted into the activity by the therapist standing the object first on her hand for the child to pick up and then on a table. Other games can be introduced, such as dropping marbles on to a helter-skelter or a sloping bagatelle board. The older child will enjoy first removing and then placing into position the pieces of an inset jigsaw. Some such puzzles have small knobs attached to each piece but if not a small bead can be fixed with a gimp pin to give a point of grasp.

These specific training activities unfortunately expect the child to use his prosthesis instead of his normal hand. This can lead to resentment if the child is asked to use the prosthesis exclusively. Use of the other hand should be incorporated into the activity, with perhaps the hand competing with the 'fingers', or part of the activity being done with the hand and part with the prosthesis.

Specific training activities should be interspersed with more general bimanual activities which can progress to include games where the 'fingers' actively hold part of the equipment. A wheelbarrow cannot be pushed with one hand so the 'fingers' must play their part by grasping one handle. Similarly they have a part to play in holding a sieve or a cotton sack in the shape of a person or animal to be filled with sand. Cups and funnels can be easily held and filled with water, progressing to tea parties as control improves. Bathing a doll and washing its clothes is another form of water play that requires two hands and can also introduce the child to the skills of dressing and undressing.

Threading is another excellent bimanual activity as it can be graded from large blocks or rings threaded on a piece of dowel, before the child is old enough to learn how to thread on a string, through diminishing sizes of blocks to quite small beads. After threading comes screwing, which can progress from screwing on to a threaded dowel to simple assembly toys using large plastic nuts and bolts. Another progression from threading is a sewing card, which can be made from a stiff Christmas card with a simple design. The two halves of the card should be pasted together to give extra body and the holes punched or pierced with a large bodkin or awl. It is advisable to trace the outline on the reverse side otherwise the young child finds it difficult to follow.

For all these bimanual activities the prosthesis plays the non-dominant role. It holds the dowel or needle for threading, the bolt while the nut is screwed on and the card for sewing.

Sometimes the 'fingers' need to be rotated in the forearm of the prosthesis so that the object is more easily grasped or used in conjunction with the other hand. To begin with this must be done by the adult supervising the training but gradually the child should be asked to turn it round himself. A good game to teach a child how to work out the correct angle consciously is to have a posting box with the slits positioned at various angles. This training should be left until the child is confident in controlling the 'fingers' and can be the purpose of a later period of training when the use of the prosthesis is being checked.

Gradually the child begins to use the prosthesis spontaneously in his free play, as he begins to find it of use.

Activities of daily living

UNDRESSING AND DRESSING

The child with one hand should be encouraged to start undressing and dressing himself at the normal age for achieving these skills. He should have very little difficulty in learning to undress and dressing should not prove a great problem. Fastenings are likely to be the main difficulty. Clothes should be loose-fitting and tight elastic at the waist of trousers in particular should be avoided as it can hinder the learning of toilet independence. If the child does have difficulty in pulling trousers up and down, loose-fitting ones with braces may help him overcome this difficulty. When putting on shirts and sweaters he should insert the arm wearing the prosthesis before pulling it on over his head.

Slip-on shoes or sandals with buckles are easier to manage than laces, but a child with a single below-elbow prosthesis should be able to tie his shoelaces by the time he starts school. Lacing and tying knots and bows should be first taught on a toy boot or practice board. The latter can easily be made by tacking two pieces of material on each side of a piece of board with different coloured tapes attached to them. These can then be tied together starting with two different coloured tapes and progressing to two which are the same. Once the process of tying a bow has been grasped (p. 84, Method 1) the child can progress to tying a shoe on the table and finally to tying his own shoe on his foot. When he reaches this stage it is important to make sure that the laces are long enough and that they have secure metal tips for threading as the child can be easily discouraged by failure.

It is probably also worth while practising buttons on a button board before attempting them on oneself. The practice board should have buttons in a variety of sizes unless several graded boards are available. A picture slotted under a clear piece of plastic provides an incentive to unbutton and see what is underneath and can be changed between visits. A rag doll with clothes incorporating the various types of fastenings provides practice in an unstructured form. The fastenings should be graded in difficulty so that the coat has large buttons and the dress or petticoat smaller ones. Hooks, press-studs and zips can also be included and a bonnet that ties with a bow.

Many parents find that the child's clothes wear into holes more quickly on the prosthetic arm than on the other. This most frequently occurs around the elbow joint and can be counteracted to some extent by wearing an inner sleeve of nylon or cotton. A good sleeve from an old shirt can be cut off and hemmed top and bottom to take elastic. This may then be put on over the prosthesis before the shirt or sweater.

WASHING AND BATHING

A child born with one hand missing will gradually learn to bath himself as he grows in independence. He should have no difficulty in achieving this skill. The child who loses a hand may need to use some of the methods described in the section for adult amputees (p. 86). The child who is wearing and using his 'fingers' for a variety of activities should be taught to wash these when he washes his other hand, using a nailbrush if necessary. This should be suitable for holding in the 'fingers' so that he can use it for scrubbing his nails.

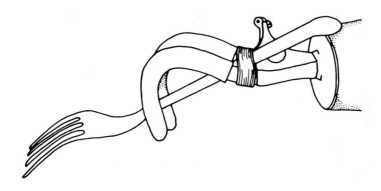

Fig. 46. Holding a fork securely in an infant split hook.

MEALTIMES: BIMANUAL FEEDING

The child should be taught how to use a knife and fork before he starts school, particularly if he is to take his dinner at school. At about the age of three children start showing an interest in using a fork to help load the spoon. This provides a good bimanual activity and is a useful introduction to using a knife and fork later. If the child is still using an infant split hook it may be necessary to put the handle of the fork underneath the rubber band holding the 'fingers' closed to keep it stable (Fig. 46). Should he have progressed to the Dorrance IOXA

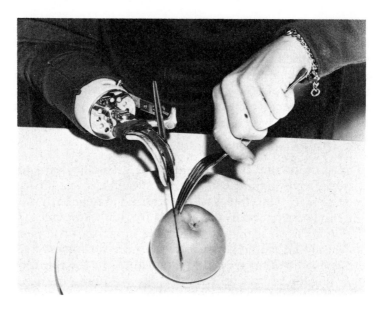

Fig. 47. A knife held in the split hook so that the handle rests on the cord lever allows for the firm downward pressure needed for cutting.

split hook the fork can be held like a pencil (see Fig. 29), with the points of the 'fingers' facing medially. Once the child has mastered the use of the fork as a pusher, he should progress to using a knife in his 'fingers' in a similar role, in conjunction with a fork in the other hand. A small child's knife should be placed in the 'fingers' in a similar way to the fork but with the points of the 'fingers' down so that the blade of the knife is at right angles to the plate (Fig. 47). Anything requiring much pressure should be cut up at first leaving only soft foods such as potato for the child to cut.

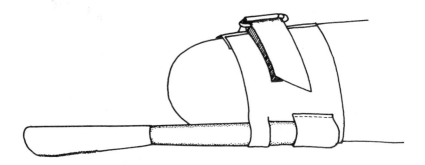

Fig. 48. A gauntlet for holding a knife.

140

The child with a long below-elbow or mid-palm absence who has not been fitted with a prosthesis will need a strap to support the handle of the fork or knife. This can be a simple strap under which the knife or fork handle is slipped, or a strap with a pocket into which the handle can be placed (Fig. 48). Whichever is decided on, the handle should be on the underside of the arm so that pressure can be exerted on the knife. The blade of the knife should be rotated 90° in the handle so that the broad aspect of the handle is against the arm. This prevents the whole knife rotating when pressure is exerted on the blade. To rotate the blade a knife with a plastic handle should be immersed in boiling water to melt the glue which then resets on cooling.

Learning to control the elbow

The child with a through or above-elbow absence is not normally given a cable-controlled elbow lock until he is about four years old. His first prosthesis will probably have a rigid elbow set at approximately 45° flexion so that he is able to use it for crawling and later, when learning to open his 'fingers' there is no loss of movement due to having to accommodate for full elbow extension. Once he has learnt to open his 'fingers' he should progress to a prosthesis with a friction elbow and lateral so that the prosthesis can be more easily positioned for use in conjunction with the other hand. Sometimes it is necessary to have a manual lock on the elbow if the child continuously knocks it into full flexion as in this position he is unlikely to be able to open the 'fingers'.

The operation of the child's cable-controlled elbow lock is exactly the same as for the adult one. The adjustment of the lock cable is very critical if the child is to learn to operate it and at first it is often necessary to tighten the cable for a practice session loosening it again afterwards so that the elbow does not accidentally come out of lock. The method of teaching the operation of the lock is basically the same as for the adult (p. 68), remembering that a child of four years has a limited span of concentration.

Preparing for school

Most parents worry about how their child will get on at school. The parents of a handicapped child are even more concerned. They realize that their child has to be able to stand up to the curiosity of other children and adults without their support and protection. They are afraid that he will either be left out or feel at a disadvantage. Starting school is a milestone for every child, so in a sense they will all be at a disadvantage. Some may have less-obvious handicaps which may be more crippling, such as shyness, insecurity, deafness or word-blindness. Their handicap may not have been recognized and so no preparation made to overcome it. The child with one hand can be prepared for school in a variety of ways.

1. Attendance at a nursery school or playgroup where he will get to know some of the children who will be starting school with him. He will then have some children who know about his limb deficiency, have seen his prosthesis and 'fingers' and have accepted him into their peer group. He will also have benefited from all the other advantages of pre-school play.

2. If this is not possible the parents can make a point of asking children who will be starting school with him to come to play with him. They should let the other children see their child both with and without his prosthesis in the normal course of play.

3. A visit to the school before the child is due to start is essential. The first visit should be without the child so that the parents can explain to the head teacher about their child's handicap and the importance of his wearing his 'fingers' rather than his hand. A second visit with the child will give him the opportunity to meet his teacher and see his classroom. Many schools now run an introductory session the term before the child is due to start school to which the mother can also go. This gives the children a chance to know each other before school starts. It is usual for children with only one hand missing to attend their local schools.

4. The therapist should make sure that the child knows how to tackle all the activities that he is likely to meet when he first starts school so that he is confident of his own ability. It is unlikely that the teacher will have either the time or the knowledge to give the child extra help with the use of his prosthesis. If the therapist is unsure of the child's ability to cope on his own she should suggest to the parents that she contact the school and either supply the relative information or arrange to visit the school. Some parents welcome this but others are afraid that this will seem as if they are asking for special treatment for their child. The parents' wishes in this must be respected. Most schools welcome information about how best to help a child use equipment with which he has been supplied.

5. A short period of training to check up on the child's proficiency with his prosthesis before he starts school is often advisable. It also makes it possible to check that the prosthesis is in good working order and fits the child, so that there is the minimum of interference with his schooling the first few months at school. The therapist should see that

the child is able to cut paper with scissors, use a ruler, tie shoelaces, eat with a knife and fork, manage coat buttons, buckles or the zip in an anorak, and take himself to the toilet for micturition.

6. At the child's next visit to see the limb–fitting surgeon a further check can be made to see that no additional problems have cropped up.

Bimanual activities for the older child

Activities of importance to a child change as he grows older and further short periods of training may be necessary, particularly when he is about to change schools or look for a job. Some children may lose a hand when older, as the result of an accident or disease, and others may require further training because earlier attempts to learn to use the prosthesis were unsuccessful.

If a child has been born without a hand and has not learnt to use a prosthesis by the time he starts school, it is probably better to wait until he reaches puberty. He is then more interested in his appearance and in achieving a higher level of skill than perhaps he is able to reach without a working prosthesis. Also he can foresee the possibility that he may need a prosthesis when he leaves school and is looking for a job. A very young child is learning to manipulate with his own hand and will develop a pattern of using hand and prosthesis quite easily, but a child who has an established pattern of using hand and stump will not easily abandon this unless there is some strong outside motivating force.

Training should be basically bimanual with the minimum of time spent on specific training in split hook control. The aim is to convince the child that a working prosthesis is going to be a practical advantage to him. Activities should be suitable for the child's age and interests and can include cooking, woodwork, metalwork, enamelling, sewing, knitting, weaving, technical drawing, Meccano, assembling kits, paper folding, model making and *papier mâché*. The use of the prosthesis for most of these activities is described in Chapter 12. Care should be taken to make sure that activities which the child will want to do at school are included. These might be any of the above as well as various sports and playground games.

Sports which are most commonly met in schools can usually be played with either the split hook, the prosthetic hand or a spade grip. Hockey, cricket and lacrosse are often easier with a spade grip, though the latter is as easy with a split hook since the stick is held off the ground. The split hook is quite efficient for holding a bow for archery and can be used satisfactorily for rounders. If the prosthesis is to be used for tennis, table tennis and badminton the ball or shuttlecock is best placed on the upturned palm of the prosthetic hand, but it is usually found easier to throw the ball for serving in tennis with the hand holding the racquet (p. 94). Netball can be played with either a split hook or a prosthetic hand but as it requires active elbow extension it is difficult for the above-elbow amputee to play. Swimming should, of course, be done without the prosthesis. Most people with one arm partly missing find it easiest to start to swim on their back or side rather than attempt breaststroke or the crawl. There is no reason why the limb-deficient child with sufficient length of arm to break the water before his head reaches it should not learn to dive. Of the playground games skipping is the most likely to present a problem. The rope tends to twist around the prosthesis through lack of wrist movement. A skipping rope with ball-bearings in the handle which allows the rope to rotate should overcome this difficulty.

Leaving school: new skills to be learnt

Most children with one hand missing progress from school to training or a job with remarkably little fuss considering the challenge it presents to them. Credit must be given to the parents, school teachers and youth employment officers for this apparently smooth transition. It is unusual for the occupational therapist to be asked for help in assessing an established limb wearer though she would routinely assess a recent teenage arm amputee. However, she is available for information and advice about the capabilities of limb-deficient children and perhaps should be used more for widening the range of occupations open to them.

CHAPTER 17

Growing Up with Both Hands Missing

A child who has both hands missing can only hold objects between his two limbs, between one limb and his chin or under his arm. All these forms of grasp have limited reach and are not always socially acceptable, but they do have the advantage of sensation. The object held or touched can be felt.

The child who has a normal shoulder joint with sufficient length of humerus to fit inside a socket can control a prosthesis in space. He is able to position it in relation to other objects which he wishes to pick up or move. He is able to operate both a cable-controlled terminal device and an elbow lock. In short he can be fitted with a useful prosthesis which is directly under his control to operate and move.

Unless a child has sufficient length of arm to use the distal ends in apposition easily and without distorting the rest of his body, he is usually fitted with bilateral prostheses. The child with one short and one long arm may be fitted on the shorter stump only while the child with bilateral below-elbow, through wrist or mid-palm deficiency may benefit more from opposition appliances with either fixed or movable opposition plates, which he may wear only when required.

A young child learns about his environment through touch so it is important that the child with bilateral arm prostheses is not made to wear them all day. Many children with this type of limb deficiency, who can and do use their prostheses extremely well, discard them for part of their childhood. The need to be able to feel and the speed and ease with which they are able to manipulate objects held between their rudimentary arms seems to outweigh any of the possible advantages that the prostheses offer. Despite this fact the ability to use prostheses from an early age ensures that the child has the choice when he is older. Once a child has established patterns of achievement without prostheses with no knowledge of the potential of the prostheses, he will find it very difficult to learn skilful use of the prostheses.

Early prosthetic training

The first prostheses should be fitted as soon as the child is approaching the age of learning to feed himself. The prostheses should have detachable soft plastic mitts covering a small wrist unit into which an infant split hook can be fitted. This will be used passively at first to hold a rattle, biscuit and other small objects of interest to the child. It is helpful if both arms are fitted identically so that it is possible to observe the child at play and using them for carrying objects from one part of the room to another. The child who has normal legs should be encouraged to use his feet for prehension so activities will have to be chosen that encourage use of the prostheses in conjunction with his feet or, when feet are unavailable, for prehension. Once the child has standing balance toys can be placed on a table so that standing and walking around the table is necessary while playing with the toys. The child can be asked to fetch objects which he cannot reach with his feet. Toys can be given to him so that he holds them between his prostheses even if he promptly puts them on the floor to manipulate them with his feet. Occasionally it is necessary to put socks and shoes on the child while initially teaching him to use his prostheses but if possible this should be avoided if he is a foot user. It is far better for the child to learn to use his prostheses in conjunction with his feet and to feel that they supplement his foot skills than to become resentful at being prevented from using his feet. It is these feelings of resentment and frustration that contribute to the child eventually discarding prostheses.

As soon as the child begins to show interest in holding objects in his 'fingers', training should start to teach him how to open them. This will proceed as for the child with one hand missing starting with the dominant arm (p. 136). Games such as Lego, picture and colour matching, inset puzzles, sand and water play all encourage control and use of the prosthesis. Bimanual activities which involve passing objects from one prosthesis to the other should be avoided at this stage as a high level of skill is required to open one set of 'fingers' without putting tension on the other.

Drawing, painting and writing

Drawing and painting are enjoyed by all children and provide an excellent medium for learning control of the prosthesis in space. Felt-tip pens are easier than crayons for these children to manage as they require minimal pressure to produce a good colour. Thick wax crayons are difficult to hold securely in the 'fingers' and thin wax crayons tend to break. Painting is ideal as the brush can be secured with a rubber band in the 'fingers' if it tends to slip or held like the fork (see Fig. 46). Washable powder paints should be used and a small quantity only put in sections of a bun tin. In this way less paint is wasted and the container cannot be tipped over accidentally. The paper can be either secured to an easel or laid flat on the table. Paintings and drawings should always be displayed for all to admire once they have dried.

Free drawing and painting should gradually give way to more specific control such as is required in drawing a house or a man. Joining dots to produce a picture teaches the older child control, but pictures are best designed by the therapist as most dotto books are too difficult for a child who is just beginning to learn to control his prosthesis. Simple writing patterns can be introduced as the child approaches school age, and writing games such as noughts and crosses, boxes and battleships are enjoyed by older and more intelligent children. Soft B or 2B pencils or fibre-tip pens should be used for writing as they require little pressure and yet have more friction on the paper than a ball-point pen.

Self-feeding

Once the child has grasped the idea of taking food to his mouth he should progress to learning to feed himself with a spoon. At first the spoon, bent to approximately 90° to allow the tip to enter the mouth, should be slotted directly into his dominant arm prosthesis (Fig. 49). The child should be encouraged to feed himself in the same way as a

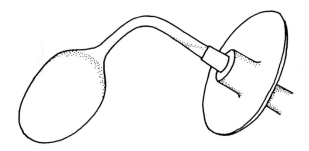

Fig. 49. A bent spoon for inserting directly in to the prosthesis.

child with normal arms learns this skill. He will need a baby plate with straight sides to assist with loading the spoon and will enjoy playing with the food. If the child is wearing an opposition plate on his dominant arm, the spoon handle may need to be padded or enlarged

147

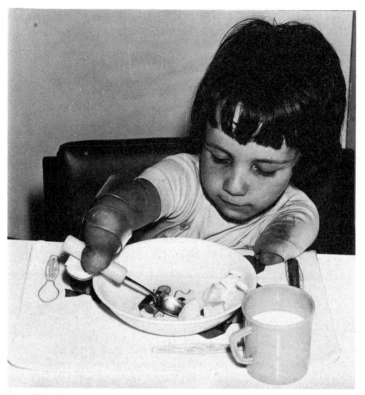

Fig. 50. Self-feeding using a spoon with an enlarged handle, held with a simple opposition plate.

with Plastazote (Fig. 50); a flat loop of metal can be soldered to the spoon so that it fits on to the opposition plate and so cannot be accidentally dropped (Fig. 51). The spoon handle should lie between the arm and the opposition plate so that the child is stimulated to hold it. Once he has mastered the art of feeding himself while holding the spoon the loop should be removed so that the child can use any spoon. Similarly the child using his prosthesis for feeding will progress from using a spoon with a tube which slips over one 'finger' (Fig. 37) to an ordinary spoon held in his 'fingers'. Picking up cutlery is the next progression (p. 111).

Most children discover that they can pick up a plastic mug in their teeth to drink. Some children manage to pick up the mug between their two prostheses but this rather depends on the length of the arms. Others pick up the mug in their teeth and then use one prosthesis to steady the bottom of the mug while drinking.

All young limb-deficient children should be allowed to feed themselves without their prostheses for at least one meal a day. Not only do

148

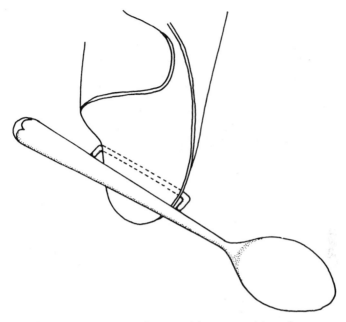

Fig. 51. A modification to a spoon for use with an opposition plate.

they need the freedom from the prostheses for part of each day but also they may need to manage without their prostheses some time in the future. The prostheses may be away for repairs or the child ill in bed. Usually it is not necessary to teach the child to do things without his prostheses. He will work out the best method for himself. This may be by holding the spoon between his two arms and swivelling it to reach his mouth, by holding the spoon between his upper arm and chin for loading and then using the edge of the plate as a pivot to bring the bowl of the spoon up to the mouth, or by using his feet (p. 162). Tea is usually the best meal for this freedom when the child is tired at the end of the day. Serious practice in using the prosthesis should be at the mid-day meal with breakfast being optional according to each individual child.

Games to improve control of the prostheses

A child learns during play and so the games appropriate to the child's age should be used for training in the use of the prostheses. Expensive educational toys are not necessary and if referred to in the text it is merely to give an idea of the type of toy. The same game can often utilize quite simple materials readily available in most homes, occupational therapy departments and schools.

149

Playing with dolls is popular with most children, boys as well as girls if they are given the opportunity. Washing the doll and its clothes is a fairly simple operation but dressing and undressing it is more difficult. Simple loose-fitting clothes should be made to go over washable dolls, with more sophisticated clothes being reserved for the more pliable dolls with a stuffed body and limbs. A large teddy or doll which has its arms 'amputated' and has been fitted with prostheses is useful to familiarize new children and their parents with the idea of prostheses. Putting the doll to bed is within the capabilities of the very young and severely handicapped child and if the cot is too high for him to reach it with his feet so much the better.

Playing shop is another game which can be structured to gradually demand more skill in controlling the prostheses; it also gives valuable practice in handling money.

Seasonal activities such as arranging flowers in a vase or making Christmas decorations and cards for various anniversaries provide variety from more traditional games. Outdoor excursions to collect leaves or plants, a scavenge hunt or a competition to see who can collect the biggest bag of scrap paper all provide an introduction to bilateral use of prostheses.

Trains and cars are always popular and can be used therapeutically if they have to be picked out of a box before being pushed around. Some wooden trains have blocks of different sized wood to load on trucks which gives additional practice in prehension. Other train sets have plastic rails which slot together; the child may need help in assembling these but should be able to dismantle them, giving practice in using the two prostheses together without expecting controlled grasp of both sets of 'fingers'.

Large tray puzzles are excellent for teaching the child to control his 'fingers' at different positions in space. At first he will only be able to manage the ones near his body but gradually he will learn that by rotating his body he is able to keep the 'fingers' closed even when he is reaching forward. If the knobs on the pieces tend to slip out of the 'fingers' a small piece of zinc plaster will provide more friction.

Many toys and games can be used for teaching the child control of his prostheses but it is important to present toys which are within the handling capacity of the prosthesis. The parts of the toys should be small enough for the child to grasp in his 'fingers' or if large have protruding pieces for grasp, such as doll's arm or knobs on puzzle pieces. Otherwise they should be suitable for grasp between the two prostheses. Flat objects such as counters should be avoided in the early stages though the child will learn later to pick them up by sliding them to the edge of the table.

Toilet independence and bathing

The older child will be able to achieve toilet independence by methods similar to the adult double arm amputee (p. 106), but the young child may need to have his clothes adapted to make this skill easier. Children with their own elbow joints should have no difficulty in pushing their pants or trousers down, providing the waist elastic is not too tight. To pull them up they may need loops at the waist to hook their 'fingers' into unless they are wearing trousers with braces. The grip of their 'fingers' will not be strong enough to maintain grasp of the material. Small boys usually find it easier to use the leg of shorts for micturition rather than take them down.

Children whose arms are absent above the elbow will need to use

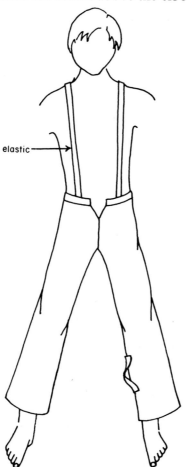

elastic

Fig. 52. A trouser modification to encourage toilet independence.

their feet for pulling down pants and trousers. A small loop of self material positioned about 12 cm (5 in) up on the inside leg seam of the non-dominant leg will make it easier for the child to hold the material with his toes when pulling down trousers. The trousers should have elastic braces and be stitched open in a short V in the centre front (Fig. 52). The underpants should be buttoned inside the waistband so that the two garments can be treated as one for dressing purposes. If the trousers are to be pulled down far enough for the child to sit on the lavatory the loop on the leg of the trouser may need to be positioned higher or a second loop stitched above the first one. However, independence for micturition should be aimed at first so this would only apply to girls wishing to wear long pants. This is an efficient and relatively easy method of coping with pants for micturition once the modifications to the clothing have been made. Children who are good foot users quickly learn to manage without the trouser loops.

Girls who wear skirts will need long loops on their pants so that they can reach them with their foot. The loops should be stitched at the side and towards the back of the waist so that the pants are pulled over the buttock (Fig. 53). The tapes can be secured to the front of the pants

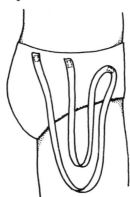

Fig. 53. One method of adapting pants so that they can be pulled down with the foot. A loop is attached to the front of the pants with Velcro to prevent it showing beneath the dress.

with a small piece of Velcro, using the prosthesis, so that they do not show below the skirt. If the child is unable to pull up her pants with her prostheses she will need to have a hook on the wall (p. 165).

The use of lavatory paper should be left until the child is a little older than is normal for independence in this skill. Children with below-elbow deficiencies should have no difficulty learning by one of the methods described for adult double amputees (p. 107), but many of them prefer to use either the heel or lavatory bowl method unless their own arms are long enough to reach. To use toilet paper on the heel the socks must be removed first. A continuous length of three or four sheets of the soft toilet paper is torn off with arms, prostheses or toes. The paper is folded in half and one end is laid across the back of the heel with the toes on the floor so that the child is able to squat down and use his heel to cleanse himself (Fig. 54). The paper can then be folded back

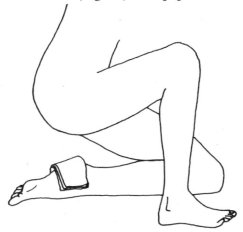

Fig. 54. Using toilet paper on the heel for peroneal cleansing.

across the soiled portion with the other foot for repeat use, and finally put into the lavatory with toes or prosthesis. The principle of the lavatory bowl method is the same in that the toilet paper is positioned and then the body moved on it. This time the paper is placed over the edge of the lavatory bowl so that one end of the paper is in the water to prevent it slipping. The paper can also be put over the seat and secured under one of the rubber knobs supporting the seat to prevent it moving. If this last method is used the paper can be positioned prior to using the lavatory so that the person only has to move sideways to cleanse himself; however, care must be taken to see that the seat does not become soiled in the process. Although these methods sound unorthodox, the fact that children prefer them to using their prostheses must indicate that they are not particularly difficult for an agile child who is accustomed to using his feet for a variety of activities.

Bimanual skills: games and everyday activities

As the child gets older and more experienced with his prostheses he will discover that he can open his 'fingers' by scapula movement rather than by pushing his arm forward. This makes it easier for him to pick up and place objects in a particular spot. It also makes it possible to learn to pass objects from one set of 'fingers' to the other, and to start using the prostheses to help with dressing skills.

By this time the child should already have learnt the bimanual skill of using the two prostheses in apposition to each other as for holding a balloon and of using one prosthesis in an active role and the other passively for either holding an object steady or for carrying something. Now the child must learn to use both hands actively even though the dominant arm takes the leading role.

USE OF CUTLERY

Using a knife and fork at meal times is a skill that most children are keen to acquire. The positioning and picking up of the knife and fork demands active use of both prostheses (p. 111). At first the child will need to have the knife positioned for him even if he has mastered picking up the fork, which he should continue to use in the accustomed arm.

DRESSING

A child born without hands should have no real difficulty in learning to dress and undress himself provided the following points are remembered.

1. He should have been encouraged to use his feet in conjunction with his arms for play activities from a very early age so that he maintains the mobility and range of movement at the hip present when a baby (p. 156). He will then be able to use his feet for dressing skills.

2. Choice of clothes should be influenced by the points listed for adult double arm amputees as most of these apply equally to limb-deficient children (p. 108).

3. Fastenings should always be positioned centre front if the child is to learn to secure them.

4. It should be remembered that the grasp which a child is able to maintain with his fingers is not very great so wherever tension has to be exerted loops should be stitched so that the 'fingers' can be hooked into these, i.e. a loop on each end of a waistband makes it easier to pull it tight for fastening.

5. A hook on the wall is a useful aid for dressing (p. 179).

OTHER BIMANUAL ACTIVITIES

There are many bimanual skills in everyday life that might be a problem for a person using two prostheses. Activities such as opening a door with a Yale lock, unscrewing a jar, opening a tin, and taking the top off a bottle are a few of these. The child should be given an opportunity to try these during training and be encouraged to attempt them at home. The more everyday activities for which the prostheses prove useful the more likely is the child to want to wear them. Crafts and hobbies such as weaving, *papier mâché*, woodwork, enamelling, stamp collecting and cooking encourage the bimanual use of the prostheses and should be included in the training programme as appropriate.

The child will usually wear and use the prostheses quite happily within the hospital or training unit but the test of successful training is when the child returns home and to his own school. Unless the adults who influence his life there are convinced that the prostheses are a good idea and are prepared to encourage the child to use them by providing suitable equipment and opportunities he will tend to discard them before he has become proficient enough to find them of value. Equally if the adults around him are too rigid in their approach to his wearing the prostheses he will rebel against them and can develop other undesirable symptoms of a disturbed and frustrated youngster. It is a tight-rope of understanding and firmness and care must be taken to ensure that the child is never penalized by wearing prostheses.

Close cooperation between the parents and the hospital or limb-fitting centre is essential so that a realistic programme for each child can be worked out. Adults accompanying the child should be present during training and be encouraged to take an active part in this so that they understand the principles behind it. Time spent talking and listening to parents is time well spent.

A clear programme should be worked out with the mother for each stage of the child's training, bearing in mind her other family commitments. Once the child starts school it is essential that contact is made with the child's teacher so that she can be kept informed of the child's current skills. The therapist can then discover what difficulties exist in the school situation. If possible the therapist should visit the school either before the child starts or soon after. The preparation and introduction of the child with both hands missing to the school environment should be the same as for the child with only one hand missing (p. 141), but it must be remembered that the teacher may never have seen a child with both hands missing before and probably will have little idea of what he will be able to do. Teachers are constantly amazed at the ability of limb-deficient children. It is always sad when a child who is able to benefit from an ordinary schooling is prevented from doing so because of ignorance.

CHAPTER 18

Growing Up with Both Arms Missing

Foot and finger training

The child without the ability to grasp with his upper limbs will develop this skill with his feet. No formal training is necessary for him to learn this skill but it can be encouraged in a variety of ways.

1. Ideally the child's feet should be uncovered at all times unless walking outdoors. If the feet are being used actively they will get no colder than the hands.

2. Once the child is a steady walker slip-on shoes should be worn so that he can easily slip his foot out of the shoe for use at any time. If socks are worn these should either have the toes open but stitched between the big and second toe to keep them down on that foot (Fig. 55) or have the sock closed but stitched between these two toes to give an independent big toe (Fig. 56).

3. Playthings should be placed on the floor and be of small enough diameter in some part for the child to grasp them between his big and second toes. Toys can be placed between the child's toes initially if he mades no attempts to pick up objects.

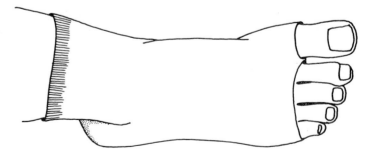

Fig. 55. A sock modification to leave the toes free for prehension.

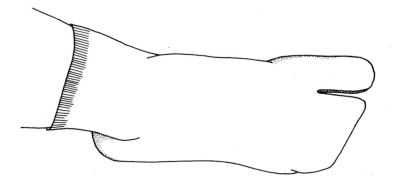

Fig. 56. A sock modification to give prehension between the first two toes.

4. Cushions should be placed around the very young child when he is using his feet at first so that if he overbalances he will not bang his head. Furniture should be removed from the immediate vicinity. Gradually the cushions should be moved away from the child so that he does not rely on them for support.

5. Different types of objects should be given to the child to play with, including everyday objects which might be out of the reach of his feet, for they are his main source of learning about texture, weight and density.

6. Sand and water play provides a useful introduction to some of the skills needed for self-feeding. A shallow tray of sand and plastic spoons and beakers are all that is needed. Water play can be in the bath (p. 168) or outdoors in the summer.

7. Children who have a single digit phocomelia should also have this uncovered for play. Later this may become important for controlling the valves or switches of externally powered prostheses. Many children develop foot dominance on the opposite side to such a digit, possibly because it is then easier for them to pass objects from foot to phocomelia. The value of this digit increases as the child learns to walk. Small objects can be carried between it and the body. In the early stages the child can be encouraged to use this digit by attaching small bells to a hair roller or practice golf ball through which he can stick his 'finger' for grasp. In this way the child begins to realize that the finger has some function.

Externally powered prostheses

These can be fitted as soon as the child has sitting balance but as

157

children rarely show much interest in using this type of arm prostheses before they have standing balance fitting is often delayed. Some children benefit from having prostheses before acquiring standing balance so that they become accustomed to wearing them. These can be non-functional and replaced with pat-a-cake powered prostheses as the child begins to show interest in holding objects with his arms. The pat-a-cake arms have a powered movement of rotation just above the elbow which brings the hands together when the elbow is positioned at approximately 90°. The forearms need to be longer than is normal for a child of this age because of the necessity to set the upper arms away from the body to accommodate friction shoulder joints. If they are not made longer the tips only of the 'fingers' will meet, making it more difficult for the child to see what he is picking up and to handle small objects. The movement is controlled by flexion and extension of the trunk with the hands coming together when the child leans forward and parting as the child straightens his back. This pattern of movement makes use of instinctive movement to reach forward to grasp. Cords attached to levers operating valves pass through rings on the waist belt and are secured to the opposite shoulder cap with a small piece of Velcro. Frequent readjustment of these cords is often necessary in the early stages, so training is better carried out without a covering garment. Groin straps will be necessary to keep the belt in position and most children need to have an elastic insert in the front of the waist belt to allow for the change in shape between sitting and standing (Fig. 57). Positioning of the gas cylinder presents problems on so young a child and it is usually best fitted to the jacket, unless the child wears lower limb prostheses when it can be accommodated in

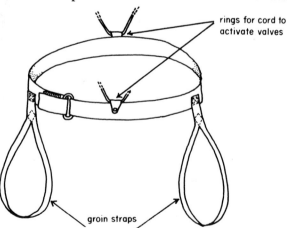

rings for cord to
activate valves

groin straps

Fig. 57. A belt for use with the pat-a-cake prosthesis powered by carbon dioxide.

the shin. Later it can be fitted to the waist belt like a gun holster but at this age it gets in the way when the child sits down.

SPLIT HOOK CONTROL

The child will graduate to a powered split hook at between eighteen months and two years. His readiness for a more sophisticated prostheses usually shows itself in a rejection of the pat-a-cake prostheses as he outgrows their limited function. At this stage dominance must be decided upon and the decision made about fitting one or two functional prostheses. Opinion has varied over the years about the best course of action. At the moment the usual practice at most centres in the United Kingdom is to fit one prosthesis with maximum function and the other with a more limited but in some cases complementary function. Two prostheses are normally fitted when the limb deficiency is symmetrical to prevent an unequal strain on the spine. The number of externally powered movements and the speed at which these can be introduced depends to some extent on the availability of control sites. The child with phocomelic digits can learn to use these to operate valves at an earlier age than it is possible to teach a child to use his acromion process for this purpose. Only occasionally does a lack of intellectual ability delay or prevent a child being able to learn to use powered prostheses.

The valves should be secured temporarily until the child has learnt to operate them as they may have to be repositioned once the split hook operation is combined with other arm or body movements. Activities to teach split hook control will be similar to those used for teaching young children to control cable-operated split hooks (pp. 136, 146). They will include activities to teach automatic control of the valves, operation of the split hook in grasp and release, and use of the prosthesis while maintaining the hook closed, as in drawing, painting and feeding. To begin with the child will have little finesse in controlling the grasp so, as this is quite strong, firm materials should be used. At a later stage more delicate objects can be handled to teach fine control.

WRIST ROTATION

Powered wrist rotation is introduced as soon after split hook control as is feasible so that the child can feed himself more easily. Otherwise a self-levelling spoon has to be used (see Fig. 60). The acromion process is most commonly used to control wrist rotation and the valve may be positioned on the same side or on the opposite shoulder depending on the total fitting plan. At some centres it is the practice to reserve the acromion on the same side for controlling a linked shoulder/elbow/wrist movement, while at others by positioning several valves around the acromion process all the controls are kept on the same side as the prosthesis which is being activated. The advantage of the latter course is that it does leave all sites on the non-dominant side available to power a complementary prosthesis, but there may be a shortage of control sites for more than one sophisticated prosthesis.

Feeding has already been mentioned as the main reason for early fitting of powered wrist rotation; it is considerably simplified by this addition. A spoon with a tube (as on the fork in Fig. 37) should be used at first to prevent the spoon being accidentally knocked out of grasp (p. 164). Other activities which can be used to teach control of this movement are turning over cards, threading discs on to dowels to make pyramids, posting boxes and any game in which the object can be presented to the child at a different angle to that in which he wishes to use it.

A period of consolidation is usually necessary after the provision of these two movements with the teaching of further movements delayed until a later date.

ELBOW CONTROL

Until this time the child has been relying on friction elbow and shoulder movements which often have to be pre-positioned by someone else. Active elbow control, either by lateral trunk movement operating on a one-pull cable elbow mechanism or as a linked externally powered movement with shoulder and wrist movement, is usually the next progression. With the one-pull elbow mechanism the elbow remains in lock until the child initiates the movement to operate it. The initial tension on the cable brings the elbow out of lock, allowing the child either to increase the angle of flexion, by increasing the tension until the desired position is reached, or to slightly release the tension, allowing gravity to lower the forearm into greater extension. A quick release of tension allows the elbow to return into lock without loss of flexion. This is an easily operated mechanism which seems to provide good control within the competence of the young child. Its disadvantages are that it necessitates the wearing of a waist belt with groin straps and that the elbow can never be free swinging. The groin straps in particular are disliked by both children and their parents, but can usually be dispensed with when the child develops a waist-line and sufficiently well-formed ribs not to be damaged by the upward pressure of the belt.

The linked shoulder/elbow/wrist movement is an integral part of the externally powered prostheses routinely fitted in Edinburgh and also of the Radius Vector prosthesis. The linked movement is designed to allow the child to reach forward to pick up objects and to bring them towards the body by activating only one valve or pair of valves. The split hook remains at a constant angle in relation to gravity and so allows a spoon or cup to be lifted to the mouth without constant readjustment of the body to prevent spilling. In Edinburgh the valve is linked to a position servo which demands constant pressure on the valve to maintain a given position. This gives the child some idea of the position of the prosthesis in space, but has the disadvantage that pressure must be maintained on the valve to maintain that position.

Activities to teach elbow control will include feeding in a more natural manner and moving objects from one level to another. A marble helter–skelter or even a sloping board to roll marbles down can be adjusted to demand a specific degree of elbow flexion. Ladder scoreboards can be used with competitive games for the older child, while drawing and painting on an upright board will encourage the child to readjust arm position in order to reach all parts of the paper.

ACCEPTANCE OF PROSTHESIS

Many children reject powered prostheses as they get older after having been proficient users when young. These children maintain that life is easier without prostheses than with them. The function of the prostheses, available at present for this degree of deficiency, gives a much cruder dexterity than the children have with their own vestigial limbs or toes. Although many admit that they would like to have arms the price that they have to pay in wearing the necessary hardware appears to be too heavy for the resulting function. Some people maintain that prosthetic hands rather than split hooks lead to a better acceptance of prostheses. This has been cited as one of the reasons for the better record of limb wearing by children attending the Edinburgh centre, and is also inferred by Nichols et al. (1968) from their study of children with multiple congenital limb deformities. At Roehampton split hooks are routinely fitted as they are felt to have greater functional capability but powered hands are available for the older child if the limb-fitting surgeon considers that the child would benefit from them. However, the substitution of hands for hooks will not make the wearing of prostheses more tolerable for the active child who finds the prostheses a hindrance to normal play even though it may make him more socially acceptable.

Activities of daily living

FEEDING

Limb-deficient children should always be taught to feed themselves without prostheses as well as with them. This has already been discussed in the previous chapter and is of even more importance to this group of children, who are fitted with sophisticated prostheses which are more liable to breakdown. The child without arms usually has the choice between foot and prosthesis, though a few can manage a special spoon with their phocomelic digit. Foot feeding is quite efficient but not always socially acceptable, so if the child can use his digit he should be encouraged to do so. Self-feeding should be started at the normal age.

The child who is going to use his foot should start feeding sitting on a chair with a back and with a seat the same height as or only slightly below the level of the table. He should have the other foot on the seat of the chair or on the table for balance. The spoon is usually held between the big and second toe with the bowl of the spoon on the sole side of the foot. To begin with he may have difficulty in getting it up to his mouth without spilling the food so self-feeding should be started with food that is reasonably adhesive (mashed potato, porridge, etc.). Some children like to rest the heel of the foot holding the spoon on the

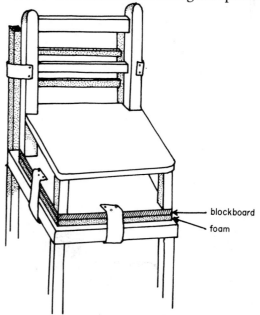

blockboard

foam

Fig. 58. A portable seat used to raise the height of an ordinary dining chair.

other leg and use this as a lever to get the spoon to the mouth. As the child becomes more proficient and his legs grow longer in relation to his body he will be able to sit on a lower chair until he eventually manages on a chair of normal height. In most homes the whole family sit round the one table for meals. To have one child having to sit so high can create problems both at home and when out visiting. One solution is to have a seat made from an old chair with the legs sawn off at the appropriate height and set on a piece of blockboard. This then has a layer of foam stuck on it to accommodate to various shaped chairs. Two straps under the seat of the normal chair and one round the back holds it firmly on most standard dining chairs (Fig. 58). The seat can easily be lowered by removing the blockboard base and sawing off a bit more of the chair legs. Some parents prefer to use an old high-chair, graduating to either a chair with raised legs or one of the commercially available tall wooden chairs for children.

The child should have no difficulty in using a fork in a similar way to a spoon but may have more difficulty in using a knife and fork together because of balance. Most children find it easier to cut up the food with a knife on its own using a rocking motion to cut the food. Although most manage with an ordinary knife, one with a curved

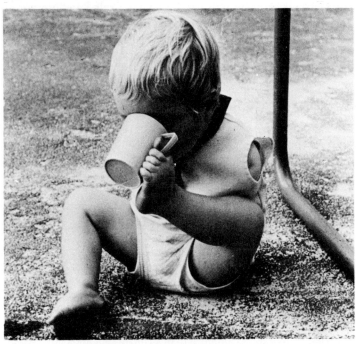

Fig. 59. A very young child has the mobility to lift a mug to his mouth using his feet.

163

blade such as a cheese knife or Nelson knife (see Fig. 73) is easier to use.

Picking up a cup for drinking requires a little practice (Fig. 59) so the child should be started with a non-spill mug. If they are standing or sitting on a low chair these children will usually opt for picking up the mug in their teeth for drinking.

Some children can feed themselves using their phocomelia and others cannot. It depends on the length, power and mobility of the phocomelia. If the child has two linked digits between which he can hold an object he has a good chance of being able to hold first a biscuit and then a spoon for self-feeding. If he has only a single digit a spoon with a handle into which he can insert the digit will have to be made. However, if the finger is weak he may be unable to control such a tool. Probably the best course is to dip the child's finger into something sweet and tasty and see if the child can be persuaded to lick the finger. If he can it may be worthwhile to persevere with activities to strengthen the finger.

Feeding with the prosthesis can start as soon as the child has control of either wrist rotation or elbow flexion. If the child has powered wrist rotation he can use an ordinary spoon, with a tube to prevent it being knocked out of alignment at first (see Fig. 37) but if he is depending on elbow movement only he will need to have a self-levelling spoon (Fig. 60). An ordinary spoon can be used with the prosthesis that has the linked elbow/wrist movement as the wrist flexes in proportion to the elbow movement to keep the spoon at a constant angle in relation to the ground. A deep plate or a plate guard (Fig. 38) will be necessary

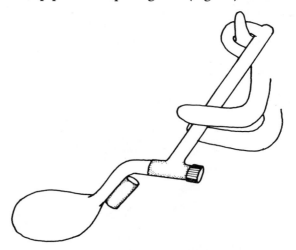

Fig. 60. A self-levelling spoon modified to fit an infant split hook powered by carbon dioxide.

initially. The child should have no difficulty in progressing from spoon to fork but he will find bimanual feeding with the prostheses extremely difficult. A fork or knife used as a pusher is possible if he has a powered lateral movement on his non-dominant prosthesis, but to cut he will have to use body movement, which is extremely difficult to do while holding the food steady with the other prosthesis. A Nelson knife (see Fig. 73) used in conjunction with wrist rotation is probably a more practical situation. Picking up a cup for drinking is much easier with the linked shoulder/elbow/wrist movement than with a cable-operated elbow. Even so the children usually then take the cup between their teeth and use their prostheses under the base only for steadying while drinking. At first picking up sandwiches and cakes is as much of a problem with powered prostheses as it is with cable-controlled ones, however, with practice the children do learn to close their split hook only partially so that a gentle grasp is maintained on the bread or cake. In the interim a sandwich holder can be used (see Fig. 43).

TOILET INDEPENDENCE AND ADAPTATION OF CLOTHING

For the child wearing prostheses independence for toilet should be first taught without the prostheses. Long trousers with elastic braces and a toe loop (see Fig. 52) are the easiest method. Boys will need to have a short V-opening in the front to make it easier for them to expose their penis; girls may need an extra loop above the lower one so that they are able to pull the trousers down far enough to sit on the toilet. Girls who prefer to wear skirts will need to have their pants adapted for pulling down with their feet (see Fig. 53) and will require a hook on the wall for pulling them up. This can be an ordinary single coat hook screwed

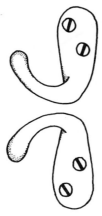

Fig. 61. The position of coat hooks for use as a dressing aid.

to the wall so that it is just above waist height when the child is squatting. She can then hook the back of the panty on the hook and as she squats down the panty will be pulled up over her buttocks. Some children prefer to use a similar method for taking down the pants so that they do not need to have loops stitched to them. The hook must then be pointing downwards so that it can be slipped inside the waist of the pants while the child is squatting and pulls down the pants as the child stands up. A pair of hooks can be positioned (Fig. 61) or a special flat double-ended hook supplied (Fig. 62). This latter device is usually supplied with a metal runner which is screwed to the wall so that the hook can be adjusted as the child grows. This method can be used by boys for pulling up trousers provided they have elastic in the waist.

Once the child can adjust his clothes for going to the toilet without prostheses an attempt should be made with prostheses. Some children find it more comfortable to have the elastic braces secured to the jacket of the prostheses with daudé studs rather than going over their shoulders and possibly interfering with the operation of shoulder valves. In this case the braces may need to be detachable from the

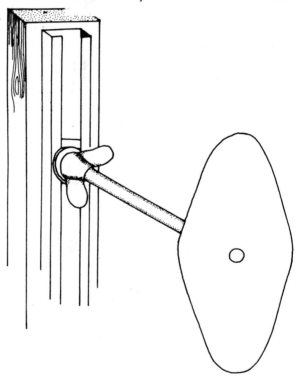

Fig. 62. A flat double-ended dressing hook on an adjustable-height runner.

166

trousers so that complete ones can be substituted when the child takes off his prostheses.

Cleansing after using the toilet is best done by either the heel or lavatory bowl method (p. 153).

Older boys who have powered elbow extension should be able to manage the zip in the front of their trousers providing a split ring or loop is inserted in the tag. Those children with a cable-controlled elbow, in which extension is by gravity, will need to use an extending trouser hook in their mouth. This hook was originally designed so that adults and children with short phocomelic arms could reach to operate their trouser zip (see Figs 65, 66). When used in the mouth a nylon mouth-piece should be added or the metal shaft covered with tubular Rubberzote or some similar material to give a better grip and to prevent damage to the teeth. Older girls will need to learn how to cope with menstruation and the various alternatives will be discussed in the next chapter (p. 182).

DRESSING

Very little other adaptation of clothing should be necessary if the child's clothes are chosen with his abilities in mind. He should be a good foot user who has maintained a wide range of hip movement. With his feet he should be able to put most garments over his head and if necessary cope with front fastenings using a combination of teeth, toes and phocomelia. Socks should be no problem as he will be in the habit of taking these on and off in order to use his feet for prehension.

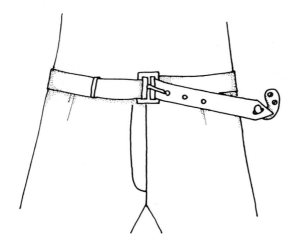

Fig. 63. Tightening a belt using a wall hook.

As they get older some children prefer to keep their feet covered when using them in public. If they wish to do this they will find the Japanese split-toe socks, designed for wearing with toe-thong sandals, impede their feet function less than ordinary socks. If these are not readily available nylon or silk socks can be stitched and then cut to separate the big toes from the others (see Fig. 56).

When wearing the prostheses these should be dressed before being put on. The shirt or dress should have a complete front opening and if closed with Velcro the child should be able to fasten this himself by pressing his body against a table or chair after positioning the material with his prostheses. The front fastening of the prostheses should be of Velcro so that it can be secured with either chin or prosthesis, and the belt buckle can be fastened with the extending trouser hook held in the mouth and tightened by using a wall hook at waist level (Fig. 63).

WASHING AND BATHING

Washing and bathing should not present great problems for these children. When very young they may need some support in the bath so that they can use their feet safely. Either a plastic bath or clothes basket can be put into the bath for the child to sit in, or if this is felt to be too restricting a plastic bath can be cut in half and secured to the base of the bath with rubber suckers to provide a bath seat. A little octopus or similar soap holder to secure the soap to the side of the bath will be a help and a long-handled bath brush will enable the child to wash his back and shoulders. Children who are habitual foot users should have some means available for them to wash their feet during the day. A firm table by the side of the wash basin, on which they can sit, is one possibility or a board across the bath to sit on while washing their feet is another. If a separate shower with a seat in it is available the child can use this provided the shower rose can be used low down. At least one school with two such children attending considered it worthwhile installing a low sink for the children to use. When drying after a bath some children find it easier to use a roller towel on a hook (Fig. 64).

WRITING AND TYPING

The very young child will have been encouraged to draw and paint with his feet. When a little older drawing and painting will have been used to teach him control of his dominant prosthesis. If he has a phocomelia with which he can grasp he will have been encouraged to use this also, to develop its ability and range of movement. These are all occasions when drawing and painting have been used as the medium for teaching other skills. When the child starts school he

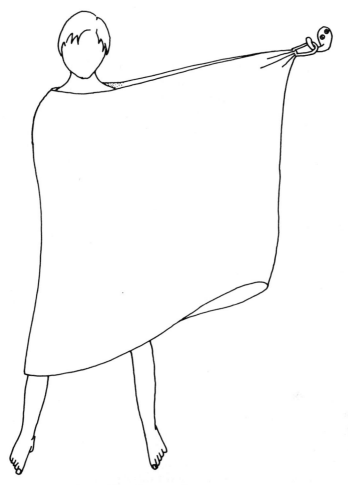

Fig. 64. Drying inside a wide roller towel.

learns to write and this becomes one of the tools of education. A decision must then be made as to how the child is going to write so that his education will not be impeded. Writing should not be used as a therapy when it should be furthering education. Usually it is wisest to let the child write in school by the method that he finds the easiest and if it is felt necessary to give him practice in writing by some other method this should be carried out specifically for that purpose at a time when his school work will not be penalized. If mouth writing is chosen a regular check should be made on the child's eyesight. It should not cause eyestrain in a child with normal vision but can make certain eye conditions worse.

Older children sometimes find that they are having difficulty in keeping up with the amount of written work required of them. For these children typing may provide a more efficient method of putting words on paper. This can be with a manual or an electric typewriter using toes, phocomelia, a mouth stick or a head stick. A manual typewriter is more convenient but many of these children have not enough strength in their toes or phocomelia digits to depress the keys fully. Portable electric typewriters provide a useful alternative.

The typewriter should be lower than the seat when typing with the toes and some children find it easier to have a book to rest their heels on to bring their feet in a good position for reaching the keys. A few children learn to touch type with their toes but many find it easier to type with a rubber-tipped pencil or dowel held between their toes. When using phocomelia the typewriter should be positioned to provide maximum reach with minimum strain on the back. For typing with a mouth or head stick the typewriter will need to be higher so that the keys can be reached without the child rounding his back. Using a mouth stick, as for writing with the mouth, can be contraindicated for children with poor eyesight. Typing should never be considered as the major means of communication until it is shown that the child is unable, or likely to be unable in the near future, to keep up with his schoolwork with writing. Typing as a vocation can be considered when the child is nearing the end of his schooling when the criteria to be considered will be largely different from those influencing the decision about typing for schoolwork.

Home and school programmes

When the child is attending a special unit or in hospital the environment is geared to give him the maximum opportunity to achieve his full potential. This is not necessarily so at home and at school, nor is it desirable that it should be so. The limb-deficient child has to grow up to fit into a world which is orientated towards people having two arms and two legs. Many occasions are going to occur when he is penalized for not having arms. He must learn to accept and overcome these difficulties if he is to fit into society. It is not being kind to a handicapped child to screen him from all difficulties during his childhood. Equally families consist of members other than the handicapped child. The parents have to share their time between all their children and the limb-deficient child must learn to take his place in that family.

The therapist must get to know a handicapped child's family if she is going to be able to help them plan a realistic home programme. She must discover from the parents what they consider to be the most important goal for their child and then discuss with them how this is to be achieved. They must plan together what are to be the immediate aims and what can be deferred to a later date. She must enlist their cooperation and support for treatment programmes and try to work out a practical way of implementing them. Involving the parents and the child in these plans will improve the chances of their success. They will feel committed and impracticalities can be avoided. Often it is possible to compromise, such as limiting dressing practice to week-ends and holidays when there is no school bus to catch. The onus for carrying out the training programme is going to fall on the parents so it is only right that they should have a hand in planning it.

The same criteria apply to planning a realistic school programme, remembering in particular that the child goes to school to be educated and not to receive training in the use of his prostheses. Most teachers are only too willing to support a treatment programme if they are convinced that it is to the ultimate benefit of the child. Usually it is only a question of ensuring that the teacher is aware of what the child is physically capable of, but sometimes active help must be enlisted. Frank discussion with the teacher about the treatment aims, with suggestions about how these might be achieved, usually leads to the working out of a realistic programme, but in the end teachers decide what the child does in school and the therapist can only ask for their cooperation.

References

Nichols, P. J. R., Rogers, E. E., Clark, M. S. & Stamp, W. G. (1968) The acceptance and rejection of prostheses by children with multiple congenital limb deformities. *Artific. Limbs*, 12(1), 1–13.

CHAPTER 19

Growing Up with Both Arms Deficient

A child who has two or more fingers on a rudimentary arm which gives him sufficient length to take these fingers to his mouth will normally reject arm prostheses as more of a hindrance than a help. He has both sensation and the ability to manipulate with his own fingers, neither of which he has with prostheses. Reach he may not have but providing he has normal lower limbs he will overcome this by positioning his body in relation to the object which he wishes to grasp or manipulate. The major area where this is not possible is when he wishes to manipulate objects in relation to another part of his body. Self-care, as typified by eating, dressing, toilet and washing, is a major problem for these children. Another area of difficulty for some of the children will be created by the very fact that they are able to lead so nearly a normal life. These children should be able to attend ordinary schools, join in most play activities and many sports. They will expect to be able to take their place amongst the adult working population. They should be able to do so but first fear and prejudice must be overcome. Physically they are capable of doing many jobs, but work-mates and employers do not always realize this.

Aids and appliances

Aids and appliances are often given to these children to help them overcome their lack of reach. There are many excellent reaching aids on the market which are primarily designed for elderly people with arthritic hips or backs, or for people who are confined to a wheelchair. These aids are designed for use with a normal hand even though it may be limited in power and often are too difficult for children with rudimentary hands to manipulate. To understand why, it is necessary to look at both the anatomy of these children and the ergonomics of controlling a lever in space.

Human beings rely on a stable shoulder joint for controlling their arm in space. Many of these children do not have a normal shoulder joint and many have no more than a miscellaneous collection of ligaments, muscle and other soft tissue connecting their rudimentary arm to their body. It is therefore not surprising that they have difficulty in controlling their arm in space and find the task of controlling an additional length in the form of prosthesis or reaching aid an almost impossible task. The longer the aid and the greater the weight at the end, the more difficult the task becomes. Man also relies on his thumb for most forms of prehension and tool handles are designed with this in mind. Most of these children do not have thumbs and so are dependent on grasp, either between fingers and palm or between individual fingers. Both of these types of grasp are relatively weak in comparison with grasp involving the thumb. Reaching aids for these children must therefore be of the lightest possible material compatible with strength and rigidity, have as much of the necessary weight near the proximal end and have a grip which is easy to grasp without the advantage of a thumb.

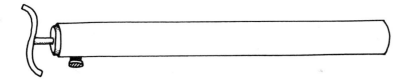

Fig. 65. A double-ended extending trouser hook (collapsed).

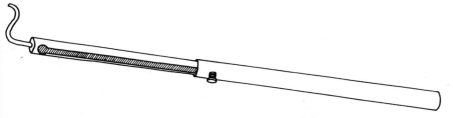

Fig. 66. A single-ended extending trouser hook (extended).

REACHING AIDS

In practice these children seem to find the very simplest of reaching aids the most useful. The reason for this is not hard to find; they are light and easy to carry around and to use; they are easily adapted to each individual child's requirements; they do not require a high level of fine coordination; and the child normally wants to achieve the goal for which the aid is designed.

Amongst the reaching aids that are found useful are extending trouser hooks (Figs 65, 66), not only for manipulating a trouser zip, for which they are designed, but also for fastening belts, pulling up trousers and pants and tightening shoelaces. The Japanese back-scratcher, which has curved fingers and is light, is an excellent tool for hooking things towards one and can be used in school when other children hold up their hand. A ruler can also be used for this purpose. A wooden dowel with a cup hook screwed into the end can be used for hooking, pulling and pushing objects and clothes. A thin dowel or rod set into the handle at right angles to the shaft makes this aid easier for some children to hold (Fig. 67). Alternative ends can be designed to fit on such a dowel providing that they do not materially increase the weight of the aid. A rubber thimble is one and a variety of these are illustrated by Nigel Ring (1972).

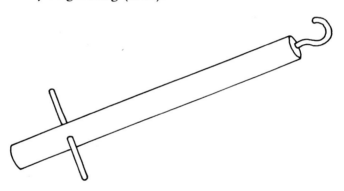

Fig. 67. A cruciate handle on a dowelling dressing aid.

FIXED AIDS

An alternative to an aid held in the hand is the aid fixed to the wall or a piece of furniture. These can be in the form of hooks (see Figs 61, 62) or designed for a specific purpose such as holding toilet paper (Fig. 68), a hairbrush (Fig. 69), a razor (see Fig. 12), or a telephone (Fig. 70). These static aids are more efficient if fixed with clamp or screws, although the telephone and razor holders do work quite satisfactorily on a weighted base. Obviously it would be more convenient if these aids were portable but repeated efforts to find a suction system that is really firm when subject to body pressure have so far been unsuccessful. The most efficient of the suction hooks is one based on an elliptical cam.

The hook is placed in position with the hook hinged upwards; as this is pulled down an elliptical cam pulls a metal disc on the concave surface of the suction pad away from the wall surface, creating a vacuum. These hooks are available commercially but the hook needs to be modified to be a useful shape for dressing.

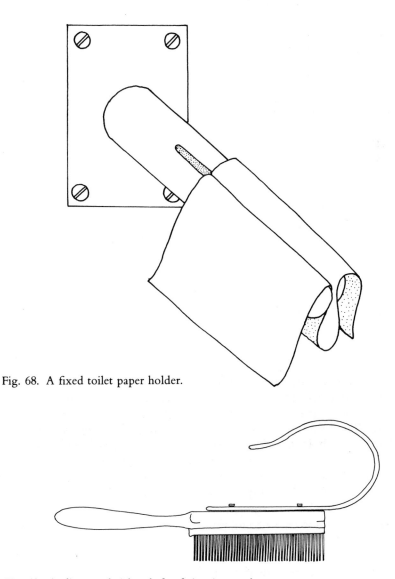

Fig. 68. A fixed toilet paper holder.

Fig. 69. A clip on a hairbrush for fixing it to a door.

175

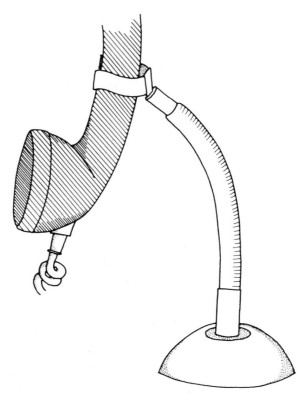

Fig. 70. A telephone on a stand can be used in conjunction with weight-on telephone buttons.

Use of feet

An aid to self-care that many of the children in this group are denied is their feet. Because they can use their hands for play, they do not naturally use their feet for prehension and are not usually encouraged to do so. They therefore lose the mobility in the hips which is present in a baby. All children with severe shortening of their arms should be encouraged to become good foot users as described in Chapter 18. They should learn to use their feet in conjunction with their shortened arms so that they develop complementary skills. Their mothers should be shown how to move the child's legs through their full range of hip movement in order to maintain the suppleness of the baby, if the child is not using his feet extensively. Prehension with the toes can be encouraged as the child gets older by competitive games with other children. Some parents are unwilling to encourage their child to use his feet in this way because they feel it accentuates the difference of their child. They want him to be as normal as possible and so encourage him to use his hands to the exclusion of his feet. This could make life more difficult for their child when he grows older. When he is very young his 'difference' will not bother him and when he is older he can choose when and where he uses his feet as an extra aid.

Self-care

USE OF CUTLERY AND DRINKING

The first of the self-care activities that any child tries is feeding. The child who has sufficient length of arm to put his fingers in his mouth will have no real difficulty in learning to feed himself in the normal sequence of development. If he has difficulty in getting the point of the spoon into his mouth he may need a curved spoon initially. The spoon needs to be light and it is usually most satisfactory to cut a spoon to the shape required out of a piece of Perspex, mould and file the bowl and then shape the handle to suit the individual child's requirements. The basic shape most often used is in the form of an S (Fig. 71). Alternatively a bar across the spoon handle to form a cross can give the child a more efficient grasp (Fig. 72) if padding is not sufficient. By the time the child is ready to progress to using a fork he should be able to manage a normal lightweight dessert fork. Light, cheap cutlery is often preferable to the more expensive stainless steel variety though not always so malleable. The ability to use a knife and fork will depend on the length and power of the child's arms. He will need sufficient

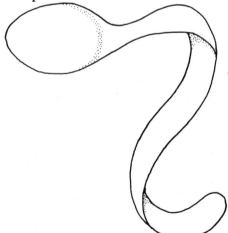

Fig. 71. A possible shape for a spoon to encourage self-feeding, when the arms are very short.

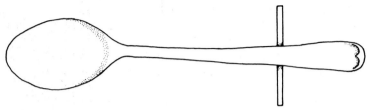

Fig. 72. A cruciate bar soldered to the spoon handle is a help to grasp when no thumb is present.

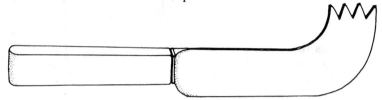

Fig. 73. A Nelson knife with a sharpened curved edge and a fork end.

length to be able to coordinate the knife and fork held in opposite hands and sufficient power to use the knife without relying on body weight for cutting. Most of the children have difficulty with cutting all but the softest foods using the standard child's or dessert knife and need a steak or small kitchen knife to cut meat or crusts of bread. Learning to use a knife for cutting may therefore have to be deferred until the child is old enough to be responsible for such a sharp knife. Some older children prefer to use a Nelson knife or cheese knife with a curved blade (Fig. 73), so that they can cut with one hand using a rocking movement. They can then utilize body power to control the knife. Many of these children, with phocomelia, choose to pick a mug up in their teeth for drinking, merely using their hand to tip the cup and support it while drinking, while those with the longer ectromelia can manage a normal mug or cup. Glass tumblers are hard to pick up without a thumb, but a wine glass is easy as the child can support the bowl of the glass on his hand.

DRESSING AND UNDRESSING

These children should be encouraged to start to help with their undressing and dressing at the normal age for achieving these skills. At this age the children are motivated to want to be independent. Many of them will need a lot of help but if they can be encouraged to take an active part, rather than stand like a doll to be dressed and undressed, they will begin to learn how to move their body in relation to the person holding the garment. They will then find it easier to use a wall hook, door handle or piece of furniture as a dressing aid. A wall hook is probably the easiest to use initially. It can be of two types as described (see Figs 61, 62). When it is to be used for removing garments on the top half of the body, such as shirts and vests, it should be fixed at shoulder level or the highest point that the child can reach with his hands, whichever is the highest. The bottom of the garment is then placed over the hook and, if necessary held there, while the body is twisted away and down from the hook so that the head can be pulled through the neck of the garment. A vest or similar garment should be laid on the bed so that the child is able to tunnel his head in through the bottom; once on the head the vest can be placed over the wall hook allowing the child to create a space within the garment by pulling away from the hook; he will then be able to manipulate his body within the garment held on the hook until he has head and hands through the correct holes. To prevent frustration garments should be loose-fitting for this exercise.

Removing pants and pulling them up with a wall hook has already been described (p. 165), but many of these children can manage pants and trousers providing they have loops to catch hold of with their

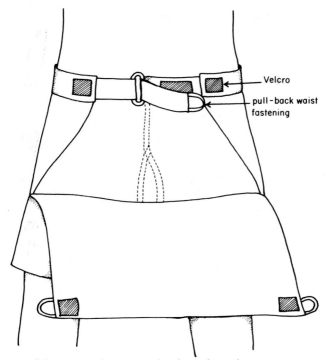

Velcro

pull-back waist fastening

Fig. 74. A modification to shorts to aid toilet independence.

179

hands (Fig. 7). Trousers can be pulled down with the toes, with the addition of a loop of material on the inside seam if necessary (see Fig. 52) and pulled up with either braces or by two loops positioned at each side of the waist. Some children's shorts and trousers have pockets each side which can be used while others have belt loops which can be re-positioned if necessary. Shorts can often be easily adapted so that the entire front panel drops down (Fig. 74). These, when worn with straight front-opening underpants, make it easier for the very young child to learn to be independent for micturition. Shorts with two side pockets should be chosen so that there is sufficient material for an overlap. Later he should be able to manage a front zip with a ring or loop in the tab either with his own hands or with the help of an extending trouser hook (see Figs 65, 66). Some people with short arms find it easier to have the fly zip extended to the top of the waist band with just a flap of material secured over this with Velcro as this does away with a tight waist fastening. Girls often only need to have short loops on one side of their pants, one to pull them down with a foot and one to pull them up with a hand (Fig. 75). If a longer toe loop is necessary this can be secured to the front of the panties with a piece of Velcro to prevent it showing below the hem (see Fig. 53).

Socks are often a problem for this group of children because so many of them are not good foot users and they cannot reach their feet with their hands. Various types of sock and stocking gutters should be tried to discover the one best suited for each individual child. However, using these aids is a tedious business and many children opt out of this activity and are prepared to accept help. Tights with a split gusset avoid the necessity of taking them down for micturition and so limits the need for help.

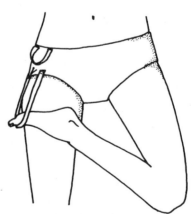

Fig. 75. A modification to the pants for an older girl with a longer phocomelia or ectromelia.

Fastenings need not present a problem for this group of children provided they are positioned within their reach. They are most likely to have difficulty if tension has to be exerted while securing a fastening such as at the waist of skirt or trousers. Loops on each end of the waistband, so that the 'fingers' can be hooked into these rather than having to grip the material, may make this easier, while elastic waists do away with any fastening. Buttonhooks may need to have extended handles with perhaps a cross bar or additional padding to improve grasp (Fig. 76). Shoes should be slip-ons.

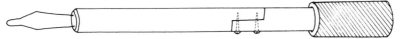

Fig. 76. A buttonhook, showing the extension and the padded handle.

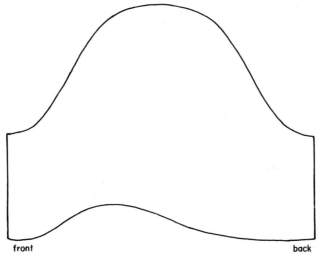

front   back
Fig. 77. A modified sleeve pattern to prevent material in front of the sleeve impeding the function of the hand.

Clothes must be chosen so as not to impede the already limited function of the arms. Children with very short arms should have coats with raglan shoulders so that the sleeves can be cut short enough in the front not to cause bunching of material under the hands; these children should wear shirts or dresses without sleeves or with the sleeves cut shorter in the front than at the back (Fig. 77). Children with longer arms should have full length sleeves cut off at wrist level or slightly shorter if they have radially clubbed hands.

As the children get older they naturally want to wear fashionable clothes with the minimum of obvious adaptation. Loops on pants are often rejected when the children start doing gym in pants and vest; a

181

possible solution is for the teacher to help the child put on an unadapted pair over the adapted ones for gym. Many parents find that it is easier to make the child's clothes than to adapt ready-made ones. Often it is then possible to include the type of fastening that the child can manage without altering the style of the garment.

TOILET INDEPENDENCE

Once the child has learnt to adjust his clothes for toilet independence he will progress to using lavatory paper. If the child can almost reach with his own hands he may only need a device to give him more reach, such as a Spontex mop over which he can place the tissue. However, most children opt for either the heel or lavatory seat method (p. 153). Other methods which have been used are toilet tongs, which were eventually hinged in the middle to make it possible to carry them in a knitting bag, a two-pronged toilet appliance on a handle and a toilet-paper holder screwed to the wall (see Fig. 68).

MENSTRUATION

Most of the girls find that the sanitary towels which fasten in the front of the pants, such as Kotex New Freedom, are the most satisfactory way for them to cope with menstruation. Alternatives are the towels with an adhesive strip up the back or ones that fit into pockets in the panty. Providing the girl can manage her own pants she should have no difficulty in coping with a normal period. A few girls are bound to have difficulties and for them a bidet may make these few days each month more tolerable. As a last resort there is always the Clos-o-mat lavatory but this should not be necessary except in exceptional circumstances.

School activities

The majority of the children in this group can and do attend ordinary schools. Generally they have no difficulty integrating into the school community. At the primary school stage their main problems are concerned with manipulation of scissors and in holding and controlling a pencil. Toilet and dressing independence can become a problem if not achieved by the time the child leaves the infant classes.

By secondary school these difficulties should have disappeared but others will take their place. More writing is expected of the child so fatigue may be a problem. Alternatives such as using a typewriter, tape recorder or speed writing may have to be considered. Accurate use of rulers and other measuring equipment becomes necessary. Practical subjects such as chemistry and cookery pose their own problems.

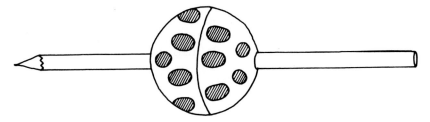

Fig. 78. A practice golf ball threaded on to a pencil may make it easier to control.

WRITING

Most children with some sort of grasp in their phocomelia do learn to use an ordinary pencil, but if this grip is very weak the child may initially need some sort of aid to make pencil control easier. A piece of soft foam taped around the pencil may be sufficient or inserting the pencil through the holes of a practice golf ball (Fig. 78) can give better control. All writing aids tend to be rejected by the children as soon as they have mastered how to control the pencil unaided and so to fabricate sophisticated pencil holders is rather a waste of time. Choice of writing equipment can make a lot of difference to these children. Pencils should always be soft (2B or B and never 2H); wax crayons are far easier to use than the hard pencil crayons; painting sticks, felt pens and nylon-tipped pens are fine, while ball-point pens require greater control. Some children can use fountain pens while others find that the nib tends to catch in the paper. The table or desk may need to be higher than for a child with normal length arms of the same age, and some of these children find it easier to write on a sloping surface rather than a flat one. One solution for the child at primary school is for him to have a sloping desk top which can be clamped on to the standard classroom table to bring the writing surface up to the correct height. This can be moved to the new classroom each year with the minimum of fuss. At secondary school this is less practical with the constant changes of classroom, but by then the child has usually learnt to accommodate to tables of different height. In the early stages of drawing and writing the child may need the paper secured to a board or the table top, but by the time he has progressed to using a book to write in most children can hold it steady with the other hand. If this persists as a problem a clipboard is an easy solution which the child can eventually learn to operate himself.

USE OF SCISSORS

To use ordinary scissors efficiently requires a thumb, not only to open and close the blades, but also to exert the necessary pressure on the blades to bring them in opposition to cut. Cheap blunt scissors are more difficult to use than the more expensive precision scissors. However, there are now several alternatives to conventional scissors

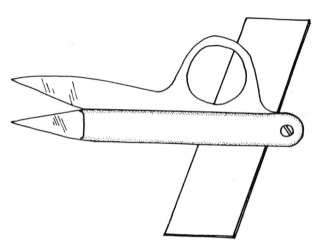

Fig. 79. Weaver's snips modified for use one-handed on a table.

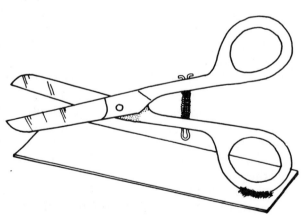

Fig. 80. Modified scissors, with a spring for automatic opening and a metal plate, for use one-handed on a table.

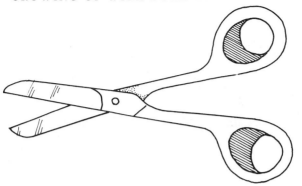

Fig. 81. Smaller finger holes in scissors prevent loss of function due to poor grasp.

for cutting. Snips are said to cut anything, have a spring opening, are safe for small children to use but may have too wide a handle for small hands to grasp. Weaver's snips are designed for use in the palm of the hand but can be easily converted for use with one hand on the table (Fig. 79). Ordinary scissors can be used similarly but will need to have a small spring inserted between the handles to keep them apart (Fig. 80). Some children can use scissors normally if the holes are made smaller (Fig. 81), while older children can use battery-operated scissors for cutting material and a razor blade set in a stand makes a useful aid for cutting threads.

TYPEWRITERS

Typing seems the obvious alternative when writing is too slow or tiring but it does have certain disadvantages for use in an ordinary secondary school. It is noisy and distracts the other children. The typewriter would need to be carried around the school by some other person if it is to be used exclusively and it needs to be stored in a safe place when not in use. An electric typewriter may be needed to achieve any speed with weak hands but can produce an additional problem as to where and when it can be used. Many of these children do in fact use a typewriter for part of their school work, but most of them use it exclusively for homework. A typewriter is certainly an aid which must be considered carefully if the child is hoping to go on to take external examinations.

TAPE RECORDERS

A tape recorder can be useful in certain situations. One science teacher found it useful for the child to record experiments on tape so that he could concentrate his physical energy on doing the appropriate drawings. It can also be used for recording notes to be written up later.

185

Speed writing can be used in this way as well as it requires less physical effort at the time, though with the disadvantage that work has often to be rewritten later.

GEOMETRIC EQUIPMENT

Rulers, protractors and set-squares are often made of plastic which is difficult to hold steady. A strip of adhesive tape stuck on the under surface will often provide sufficient friction to enable the child to hold it steady. If this is not sufficient or the child's non-dominant arm is not long enough to reach and hold, a mouth-stick, made from dowel or plastic rod with a rubber thimble on the end, will provide an additional point of pressure. Some children prefer to overcome this problem by using the pencil in their mouth and holding the ruler or set-square with their dominant hand. In chemistry a test-tube holder will often enable the limb-deficient child to take a more active part in an experiment, although a teacher's hesitation in allowing any handicapped child to handle potentially dangerous chemicals must be appreciated.

KITCHEN EQUIPMENT

The availability of electrical gadgets in the kitchen makes it easier for the handicapped child to take an active part in cookery. Using the oven is probably the most difficult as so many of these children use their chin or body to stabilize their arms when lifting or carrying. One solution is to have a small trolley of the same height as the oven shelf most commonly used. The cake tin or dish can then be placed on a baking tray on this trolley, pushed up to the open oven door and slid into the oven. When cooked the baking tray can be pulled out on to the trolley with a pair of kitchen tongs or similar reaching tool. A casserole can be served from this position and cakes left until cool enough to handle safely.

CRAFT ACTIVITIES

Woodwork and metalwork are two other practical subjects for which special arrangements may need to be made. Handles of tools may have to be modified so that they can be grasped more easily and bench clamps used for processes where holding is the normal practice. Even if projects have to be simplified the children should be given the opportunity to take part in these practical subjects. They will often surprise with their ingenuity at overcoming what seems to be an insurmountable problem.

SPORT AND RECREATION

Education is not, of course, confined to the classroom and these children will want to take part in sports and recreational activities. Their handicap for some games will be so great as to make the game meaningless to them, but there are sports in which these children can compete on near-equal terms. Swimming is one of these and football another. Riding is enjoyed by some but is less easily available in a normal environment. For the musical child there are several musical instruments which can be within their capabilities. The glockenspiel, zither, melodica, trumpet, drums and other tympani are all possible instruments for the child to try.

There are also many hobbies in which he can take a full and active part: stamp collecting; art in many of its various forms; gardening, either indoor or in a raised bed; and many crafts such as weaving, basketry, beadwork and tie-dyeing. Obviously there are going to be activities from which he feels excluded and these will always seem the most desirable. Sometimes they can be brought within the capabilities of the limb-deficient child by adapting the equipment. A bicycle can usually be modified so that the child can safely ride it. High handlebars can be angled towards the saddle to bring them within the child's reach and a back pedal brake involving the replacement of the rear wheel can be used. These are available from Raleigh Cycles despite what local retailers may say. Stabilizers can be fitted at first to give the child more confidence. Legally a bicycle should have two independent brakes so the front brake should be positioned on top of the handlebar so that the child can use body weight to engage it. Often equipment designed for other handicaps can be used to advantage. A fishing rod holder for the man with only one useful arm, that steadies the rod in a sling around the body, can be adapted for use by a child with short arms. If a child really wants to join in a sport or hobby he should discuss it with someone in a position to help him realize his ambition. This might be his parents, doctor, occupational therapist, social worker or teacher. Every avenue should be explored before abandoning the idea.

References

Ring, N. (1972) Miscellaneous aids for physically handicapped children. *Interclin. Info. Bull.*, *XII(3)*, 1–12.

CHAPTER 20

Growing Up with Three or Four Limbs Deficient

The child born with one or two limbs severely shortened or missing becomes remarkably efficient despite their absence. He learns to use his prostheses or to compensate by using other residual abilities. To have both legs and both arms affected more than doubles the handicap. It denies the child the opportunity to develop the function of the other limbs to help compensate for his loss. The child born without hands develops prehension with his feet, while the child with absent or deformed legs can use normal arms for balance and mobility on crutches or in a wheelchair.

Some children with three or four limbs deficient can and do wear and use prostheses, though few tolerate wearing four artificial limbs at the one time.

Sitting balance and early walking

Most children with four limbs severely shortened have difficulty in learning sitting balance. The provision of a sitting socket or 'flower-pot' (Fig. 82) is essential if the child is going to have the opportunity to develop normally. This socket can be made of plaster of Paris or plastic and should extend to the iliac crest and be made to fit over the child's nappies. It should be mounted on a board which can be placed on the floor or be strapped to a seat as required. As soon as the child begins to show an interest in trying to move this socket around on the floor, rockers should be placed under the board so that the child starts to learn the movement that he will need to operate his swivel walkers. Swivel walkers give those children without stable hip joints the opportunity to move freely around a limited area. They have many built-in disadvantages when viewed as lower limb prostheses, but for the very young child they have the supreme advantages of being easy to control and requiring no conscious balancing as they are designed to stand on

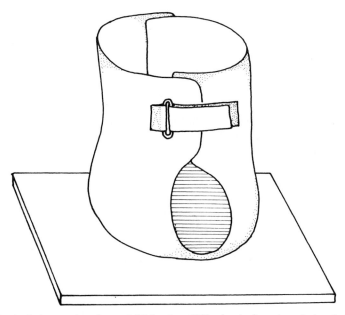

Fig. 82. A sitting socket for a child having difficulty in learning sitting balance.

their own. Their disadvantages are that sitting down in them is uncomfortable even though some models do have hip joints and locks, trousers have to be specially tailored to fit over them and they are very slow and only efficient on a smooth non-carpeted surface. However, they illustrate perfectly that when a piece of equipment is designed to fulfil a child's dominating need at a particular time, it will be accepted and can be used by the child as long as it satisfies his current need. All the very young children who are fitted with this type of lower limb prostheses, at an age when they are highly motivated to walk, accept and enjoy using their swivel walkers. As soon as other needs become more important and they begin to find the limitations of the swivel walkers frustrating they start to reject them in favour of some other form of mobility which allows them to fulfil their current needs. Some children can and do transfer to more conventional lower limb prostheses for a time, but eventually most four-limb deficient children opt for mobility in a wheelchair with costmetic legs for social occasions.

Upper limb prostheses

When externally powered prostheses were first fitted many people felt that they would be more readily accepted by the four-limb-deficient child than the child who had normal lower limbs. It was thought that the four–limb–deficient child had no alternative means of prehension while the child with normal legs was already showing himself to be a proficient foot user. Early experience did seem to support this view. Initially those children with bilateral upper limb amelia and without normal lower limbs seemed to find their arm prostheses more useful than did those children who could use their toes easily for prehension. However, as the children started to tackle more skilled activities they began to find that their mouth or rudimentary feet were more efficient than their upper limb prostheses. The development of the prostheses did not keep pace with the needs of the children and upper limb prostheses began to lose their cost-effectiveness. Of the four–limb–deficient children, those with bilateral upper limb amelia persisted with upper limbs after rejecting lower limbs, while those with upper limb phocomelia discarded upper limbs first. Upper limb prostheses seemed to have little to offer the child with some hand function despite his problems of reach aggravated by lack of mobility and poor balance. An additional factor which must affect the child's acceptance of prostheses is the restriction imposed by wearing two or more prostheses which each encase a quarter of the body surface. The effort involved in controlling lower limb prostheses combined with the lack of skin surface for heat loss could only aggravate the situation. Of eight children originally fitted with both upper and lower limb prostheses at Roehampton only one child still wears conventional lower limb prostheses and two different children still wear their upper limbs, both of which are Radius Vector gas-powered prostheses. Three of the children have cosmetic lower limbs for use when they go out. All of these children were originally fitted as out-patients before any specialized units had been set up. Four–limb–deficient children born subsequent to the Thalidomide episode have the opportunity of attending one of several specialized units in the United Kingdom. Here it is possible to have an integrated approach to the child's habilitation. Prostheses can be supplied as and when they are an aid to the child without the parents feeling that they have failed because their child will not wear them. Other aids to independence can be tried and training concentrated on making the maximum use of the child's residual abilities.

Development of skills

Children with all four limbs affected have so many skills to learn that it is sometimes difficult to know where to start. There is a temptation to overload the child by trying to teach him too many skills at once. Close cooperation between the various therapists involved is essential so that training can be programmed to dovetail rather than run concurrently. The normal stages of development can be used as a guide but should not be followed slavishly. If one skill is easier to acquire because of the nature of the handicap than another progress in the first may well outstrip the normal to the detriment of the second. However, eventually the child's urge to achieve in the more difficult area will help him to catch up. Experience tends to show that it is better to wait for some indication of the child's interest before giving a skill more than cursory attention. Certainly a very young child who has just learnt to walk has little interest in improving manual skills until he has mastered this new art of locomotion. Continuous training does not seem to markedly improve the child's function. Short spells of training interspersed with periods of consolidation often achieve a better end result, provided the adults supervising the child understand what has been achieved and how to ensure that the child makes use of what he has learnt. The difficulties of carry over at home and at school have led many therapists to favour special schools for these children so that the best therapeutic climate can be maintained. However, it must never be forgotten that the child's handicap is only one part of a very complex young person learning to adjust to the society in which he lives, and as such must not necessarily take priority over other educational and social factors which can influence the choice of type of school.

Maximizing residual abilities

In the past prostheses have not been a great asset to these children but the future can be different. New developments are continually being made and so assumptions that the child is necessarily better off without prostheses should not be made. However, whether they are used or not he will need to develop the maximum function possible in his vestigial limbs. These are one of his main channels for learning about his environment, for it is with his fingers and toes that he will feel the texture of things, learn about their weight and how they work. He may need these digits to work valves or switches on his prostheses and he may want to use them for feeding himself and writing. He should be encouraged from birth to become aware of their potential. If he cannot see them they should be handled and talked about. Small bells can be attached to them so that their movement produces some desirable effect. If the child has two or more digits he should be encouraged to hold light objects between them which should be long enough so that the child is able to see what he is holding. Strips of foam, a ring rattle, which is easier to grip than a conventional shaped rattle, wobbly and hanging toys all encourage the child to reach, move and grasp.

Many limb-deficient children make use of their mouth for feel, prehension and manipulating tools. Little instruction in learning this skill is needed though care should be taken to see that the child does not abuse his teeth while they are still developing. Orthodontic specialists would like these children to use specially moulded mouth pieces for holding such objects as pencils and paintbrushes but the children tend to find that they are clumsy and limit their capability. Invariably they get lost. In fact the children only use their teeth to steady the pencil, controlling it with their lips and tongue, so it is easy to see why they reject the mouth pieces. They also use their lips to transfer an object from one phocomelia to the other if their arms are not long enough to reach across the midline. The very young child with complete absence of arms should be shown how to use a paintbrush in his mouth or on a head band (Fig. 83), for with good head control both skill and speed at writing can be developed.

Head control can also be used for typing and for extending the child's reach into space. The Dynamic Enabler developed in the occu-

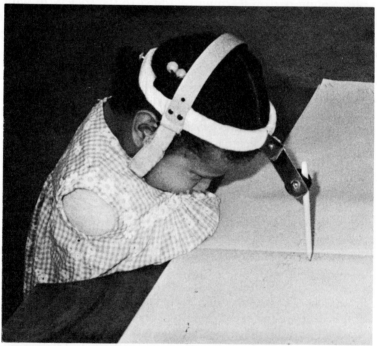

Fig. 83. Drawing using head control. (*By kind permission of the Medical Superintendent, Groote Schuur Hospital, Cape Town*)

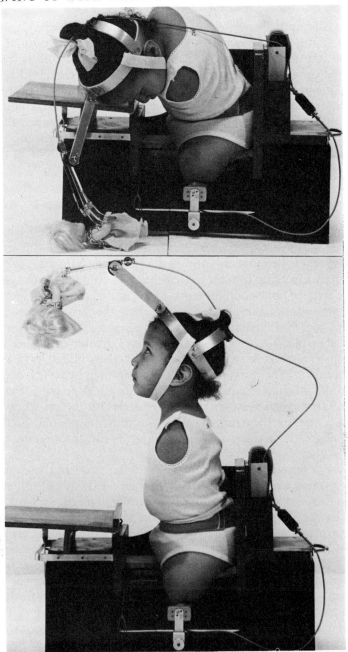

Fig. 84. Using only her limb bud to control her dynamic enabler, this child without any limbs can reach into space to pick up and examine her doll. (*By kind permission of the Medical Superintendent, Groote Schuur Hospital, Cape Town*)

193

pational therapy department of Groote Schuur Hospital, Cape Town (Schaif et al. 1976) shows how the child whose only vestigial limb is one toe can use this to operate a micro-switch controlling a gripper mounted on a head band (Fig. 84). With this aid the child is able to reach and grasp without having to wear sophisticated upper limb prostheses. The child's own proprioceptive sense is used to control the gripping device in space. When the child is older this type of aid may become unacceptable because of its rather bizarre appearance, but by then wearing and operating a more sophisticated upper limb prostheses may be more feasible.

Mobility

The conventional self-propelled wheelchair with two large wheels and two castors or small wheels cannot be controlled by this group of children unless extensively modified. One such chair was successfully adapted by lowering the seat so that the child could reach the large rear wheels with his phocomelic arms. He was able to propel and control the chair indoors but needed help when the ground was uneven. Battery-operated chairs provide a more satisfactory solution as they enable the child to go outdoors and travel greater distances without becoming fatigued. Usually those electric chairs which have a remote control box are the most suitable as this can then be positioned to suit the individual child's requirements. Modifications to the controls may be necessary when they are to be operated with the prosthesis or the toes. To operate the controls with the toes the control box can be positioned beneath the chair seat with the joystick protruding through a slot in the seat.

As well as modifying existing electric chairs to suit these children's needs several have been designed with their needs specifically in mind. One of these is a standing chair with a powered platform which can be raised by the child once he has mounted it. Once the platform is clear of the ground the vehicle can be propelled by the child at two speeds both indoors and outside on level pathways. The vehicle is designed to allow a child who can walk short distances indoors to move from one room to another at a reasonable speed without becoming too tired. It fulfils this need but is too clumsy to be used other than in the broad corridors of the special school or hospital. A chair more suitable for indoor use is one where the seat is mounted over the battery with a rail around for security. It is very mobile and designed to be used in congested areas such as a classroom or private house. It has difficulty in coping with uneven surfaces as the wheels are small but otherwise is a useful indoor chair and much liked by the children. Another chair attempted to overcome the difficulty these children have of reaching things and of getting on and off their chairs. The chair has a seat which can be raised from floor level up to table height and can be locked at any height. The chair can then be propelled by the child and though it looks clumsy its overall dimensions are no greater than the average power-drive wheelchair. This chair is extremely popular with the children. It not only gives them independence to reach objects at various heights, the ability to get on and off the chair on to the floor, bed, lavatory or another chair, but also they are able to raise themselves to talk on the same level as those able to stand. Probably the biggest disadvantage is transporting the chair from one venue to another as it is not collapsible and requires a van to accommodate it. All these experimental vehicles have had their teething troubles but do illustrate how it is possible to design a practical and acceptable piece of equipment if the child's needs are analysed rather than the able-bodied adult designing what he thinks the child should need.

The mobility aids discussed so far have been to meet the needs of the child with very short limbs but many children with long phocomelia or ectromelia of all four limbs can use prostheses indoors but need alternative mobility outside or when in congested areas. When very young, these children get around very well on the floor but as they grow older this becomes less acceptable and is never very practical outdoors. A tricycle and later a small bicycle can be the answer. Pedals can be built up with straps or even whole shoes attached to them. A spring-assist from the pedal to the handlebar will not only keep the pedal up the right way when the foot is not on it but also helps the pedal on its upward travel. Handlebars can be realigned and alternative grips fitted if necessary. A back pedal brake or a fixed wheel in the case of the tricycle is usually advisable, though some children can manage a handbrake if it is positioned above the handlebar so that downward pressure is used to operate it. The great advantages of tricycles and bicycles over wheelchairs is that they are normal play equipment for children and so play down the limb-deficient child's difference from his more complete friends. Other play equipment can often be made use of to give these children outdoors mobility in which they can safely compete with their friends. If they are unable to operate lever- or pedal-controlled vehicles there are various battery-operated cars and go-carts available. If none of these is suitable it is usually worth approaching a local technical college or university for help in adapting the most appropriate of those available. These adaptations have to be tailor-made to suit each child's abilities as the tolerance between success and failure is very small when physical skills are limited.

Clothing

When all four limbs are severely shortened or missing the available skin area for heat loss is drastically cut. It is therefore essential that the child should not be overdressed in clothes made from non-absorbent materials. These children do not feel the cold and are usually more comfortable if clad only in cotton vest and pants with cotton or light wool top garments. Synthetic materials should be avoided.

As well as making the children uncomfortable excessive clothing will restrict their use of their shortened limbs. Parents naturally want their child to look as pretty and as acceptable as possible and may be tempted to choose clothes which partially conceal deformed limbs. This is all right if the child can discard the covering material easily, as with a cape, but frills, sleeves that are too long or skirts that hamper the child's mobility can severely restrict function. Simple designs using pretty materials will enhance the child's appearance and yet allow him to make maximum use of his vestigial limbs. Often it is more satisfactory to make the child's clothes rather than attempt to alter ready-made garments. Points to consider are as follows:

1. All limbs and digits should be left free for use even if they appear to have no function.

2. If arms are very short, sleeveless garments are often preferable. If garments with sleeves are chosen they should be cut off shorter in the front than at the back (see Fig. 77), so that the material does not bunch under the hands.

3. Pants for girls are often better made with short legs with elastic rather than cut away, except when only a single digit is present. Children with total amelia of arms or legs can have the arm or leg holes sewn up if it is preferred.

4. Clothes should be made of tough washable materials which will stand frequent contact with the floor.

5. Rolling and hitching on the floor tends to encourage clothes to come apart at the waist so there should be ample tuck-ins and overlap. Dungarees and pinafore dresses avoid this problem.

Initially clothes should be made to maximize residual function, avoid heat retention and improve social acceptability, but later independence for toilet and dressing skills will have to be borne in mind. Those parts of Chapters 17, 18 and 19 which are appropriate can be applied to these children provided that one remembers that the child's mobility and balance will be severely impaired.

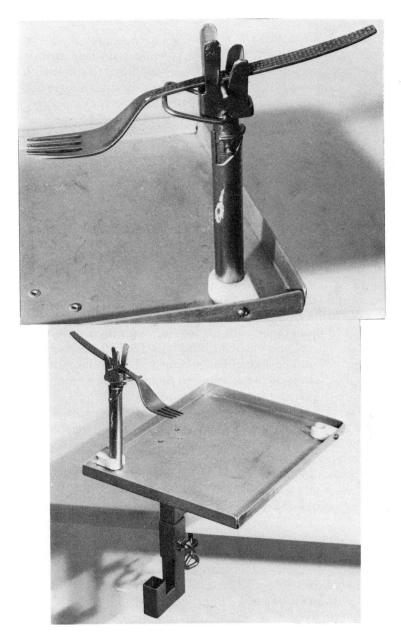

Fig. 85. A rotating feeding device with the fork in position. Plans are available from the Leon Gillis Unit, Queen Mary's Hospital, Roehampton, London.

Activities of daily living

Some degree of independence should be possible for these children, though many of them will remain dependent on help from others unless their environment can be radically modified to suit their handicap. Some local authorities are now building flats and houses designed for use by those confined to wheelchairs, while others are prepared to modify or build on to existing accommodation. The main areas of difficulty will be in the bathroom, in access to the house, in negotiating stairs and in mobility outdoors.

Many of the problems referred to in earlier chapters will, of course, be present, some of which can be solved in similar ways. Attention will be focused here on additional areas of difficulty highlighted by the multiple handicap.

1. *Self-feeding*. The child with amelia of the upper limbs coupled with amelia or short phocomelia of the lower limbs cannot learn to feed himself by any of the methods previously described in Chapters 18 and 19. When he is fitted with prostheses he will learn to use these but he should have an alternative method of self-feeding. One of the parents of such a child devised a very efficient rotating spoon which can be picked up in the mouth for loading with food, then placed by the child on a pivot and pushed round with the child's chin or tongue so that the food can be conveniently removed from the spoon or fork (Fig. 85). The whole device is made so that it can be clamped to most tables and is adjustable to the correct height.

2. *Independence for toilet*. Few four-limb-deficient persons can manage to get on and off an unmodified lavatory or to use toilet paper. The Clos-o-mat toilet is ideal for these people and should be sited so that the handicapped person can manoeuvre his chair close to it for transfer. The toilet should be set to the same height as the chair and rails provided each side for security. Forward transfer is the easiest if you have no legs and does away with the necessity of having movable side rails.

3. For *bathing* either a hoist over the bath or a shower cabinet with a slatted seat, filling the entire space and at the same level as the chair being used, is necessary. The slatted seat can be hinged so that other people can use the shower when it is folded away. The standard slings provided with most hoists are not usually suitable and it is better for these children to have a seat attached to the hoist. This can be of moulded plastic, slatted wood or be a wooden lavatory seat with rubber door stops underneath. The latter was fitted for one child so that it could be used for both the bath and the lavatory. The hoist will have to be electrically powered if the child is to operate it himself.

4. If it is necessary for these children to negotiate stairs a lift needs to be installed. The choice is between a stair lift or a vertical lift. A stair lift can only be fitted if the flight is continuous without bends and has sufficient space at the top and bottom for getting on and off. A vertical lift can be fitted in a private house without a lift shaft with the base of the lift forming the ceiling of the downstairs room when it is raised. Most lifts are electrically powered but there is one vertical lift which operates by counter weights.

5. Access in and out of buildings can be a problem unless the building has been designed with access for the handicap in mind. Most houses have a step or sill at the door and many have a flight of steps outside. Although these can be altered fairly easily in the handicapped person's home they continue to provide a barrier to mobility elsewhere. Portable ramps are available but these necessitate another person positioning them for use.

6. Although it is now possible to take some types of electric chairs on the street, it is usually not practical for a severely handicapped person to do this unescorted. Many of these chairs will not negotiate kerbs and their range without recharging is limited. Outdoor vehicles have been modified and this would seem a better solution. Initially these will probably be battery-operated but eventually it is hoped that safe modifications can be done to petrol-driven vehicles so that four-limb-deficient persons will not be restricted by the limited range of electrically powered vehicles. When provision of an outdoor vehicle is being considered access to the vehicle must be provided for. An integral garage with ramped access from the house would seem ideal. If transfer directly from the indoor chair to the outdoor vehicle is not possible a hoist may have to be considered. When this is necessary the handicapped person is going to be confined to his vehicle until he returns home. A possibility which is being explored is for a vehicle into which the indoor electric chair can be driven and then locked into the driving position. This could provide easier mobility for many handicapped people but perhaps by sacrificing the feeling of normality experienced when sitting in an ordinary car.

References

Schaif, A., Abrahams, D. & Best, A. C. H. (1976) The dynamic enabler. *Occup. Ther.*, *39(8)*, 205–7.

CHAPTER 21

Preparing for the Future

Parents are naturally concerned about their children's future. They want them to have the best opportunities and yet wish to protect them from the cruelties of a sometimes unthinking society. Children have to learn to stand on their own feet. Few children avoid being hurt even if they appear to have been born with all possible advantages. Protecting them to the point of stifling their initiative does not help them. During their childhood they should be prepared for independent lives, learning to not only feed, dress and care for their personal needs, but also to become emotionally and socially independent.

Limb-deficient children will have the same problems of growing up and learning to adjust to the society in which they live as do physically complete youngsters, but they are also going to feel that their handicap is to blame for their failures. It is going to be difficult for them to realize that other young people suffer as they do and that failure to win acceptance by one's peers may have nothing to do with having a physical abnormality. An interest in others and a sunny disposition is more helpful to integration than the ability to achieve skills or be physically complete. However, young people do want to excel and so it is wise to encourage those skills that a person has for which his disability is not a handicap. The person with normal legs can dance, skate and ski regardless of the length of arms or degree of manual dexterity, while the person with normal manipulative ability may be able to excel at model making, art or playing a musical instrument. He is then able to contribute to a social occasion and enjoy being part of a community activity.

It is always difficult to discuss in a general way career prospects for specific children who have a variety of handicaps and a wide range of skills and potential abilities. Perhaps the most useful thing is to remind parents, doctors, teachers and therapists that handicapped young people should not be slotted into what is considered a good job for that handicap. They are individuals with preferences and potential skills beyond the purely physical ones concerned with manual dexterity. An attempt should be made to discover each child's aptitudes and aspirations and to see whether it is possible for him to pursue his chosen career or a related one. There are few careers closed to the child with only one limb missing providing he has determination to succeed and the other necessary abilities. The choice is more restricted when two or more limbs are involved but need not be limited to the traditional jobs for the handicapped such as car-park attendants and lift operators. People with both arms severely shortened or absent are successful draughtsmen, switchboard operators, typists, clerks and receptionists, while others have found satisfying careers in education, law, accountancy and the church. Preconceived ideas about the potential abilities of a limb-deficient person should never cloud the search for a suitable and satisfying occupation. Sometimes an educational psychologist can help a young person discover hidden talents which may open up opportunities beyond those normally considered as within the capabilities of a handicapped person.

Many young people are keen to start earning as soon as they leave school, but it is worth remembering that a training gives the handicapped person an advantage over the untrained applicant for a job. As well as all the normal training schemes available in the United Kingdom to youngsters leaving school, handicapped young people have several special colleges for further education. Some of these give a general training while others provide specific courses. The Youth Employment Officer or the Disablement Resettlement Officer at the local Employment Services Agency will be able to provide all the up-to-date information on these colleges as well as other training courses.

Leaving school and entering the world of employment can cut a young person off from the security and unquestioning acceptance of those who have known him since early childhood. Suddenly he feels that he is on his own with his difference constantly brought up before him by the reaction of those around him. He needs the unwavering support of his family and friends at this time. Organizations such as PHAB, the Association for the Physically Handicapped and Able-bodied young people which is affiliated to the National Association of Youth Clubs, can help the handicapped person realize that he is not alone with his disability.

Independence may seem to be an impossible goal for some of these young people but, with equipment and working conditions individually designed, even the most severely handicapped person can have a measure of independence. Rearranging furniture, widening doors, eliminating steps, fitting a shower or lever taps can all in individual cases solve an independence problem. More sophisticated equipment such as POSSUM controls, variable height electric chairs and individually modified cars may open up a whole new field of activity for the severely handicapped person. However, all of this may be of only limited value if the person remains emotionally dependent. He will never be able to exploit either his talents or his equipment if he is unsure of his own psychological ability to cope with situations that may arise. To give him confidence he must be shown that independence is possible and reassured that he will not be rejected once he is no longer dependent.

Every individual has some skills which can be developed to give satisfaction and pleasure to others as well as themselves. Few limb-deficient persons have any impairment of speech, sight or hearing. All have some physical skills, however limited. Most have at least average intellectual capacity. These abilities can all be developed so that these young people have something to contribute to society. They must be encouraged to think of themselves as potentially independent people for they have the right to expect to be able to earn their own living, marry and raise their own children. They may not all be independent in body but they can all be independent in thought.

Index

Italic figures indicate an illustration